OUR UNSYSTEMATIC
HEALTH CARE SYSTEM

OUR UNSYSTEMATIC HEALTH CARE SYSTEM

Fourth Edition

Grace Budrys

ROWMAN & LITTLEFIELD
Lanham • Boulder • New York • London

Published by Rowman & Littlefield
A wholly owned subsidiary of
The Rowman & Littlefield Publishing Group, Inc.
4501 Forbes Boulevard, Suite 200, Lanham, Maryland 20706
www.rowman.com

Unit A, Whitacre Mews, 26-34 Stannary Street, London SE11 4AB,
United Kingdom

British Library Cataloguing in Publication Information Available

Library of Congress Cataloging-in-Publication Data

Budrys, Grace, 1943– , author.
Our unsystematic health care system / Grace Budrys. — Fourth edition.
  p. ; cm.
Includes bibliographical references and index.
ISBN 978-1-4422-4846-5 (cloth : alk. paper) — ISBN 978-1-4422-4847-2 (pbk. : alk. paper) —
ISBN 978-1-4422-4848-9 (electronic)
I. Title.
[DNLM: 1. Delivery of Health Care—United States. 2. Health Care Reform—United States. 3.
Health Policy—United States. 4. Insurance, Health—United States. W 84 AA1]
RA395.A3
362.10973—dc23
2015015106

∞ ™ The paper used in this publication meets the minimum requirements of
American National Standard for Information Sciences Permanence of Paper
for Printed Library Materials, ANSI/NISO Z39.48-1992.

Printed in the United States of America

CONTENTS

LIST OF ACRONYMS: A RECIPE FOR ALPHABET SOUP

AAMC	American Association of Medical Colleges
ACA	Affordable Care Act
ACP	American College of Physicians
ACS	American College of Surgeons
AHA	American Hospital Association
AHRQ	Agency for Healthcare Research and Quality
AMA	American Medical Association
ANA	American Nurses Association
BLS	Bureau of Labor Statistics
CDC	U.S. Centers for Disease Control and Prevention
CHIP	Children's Health Insurance Program
CIA	U.S. Central Intelligence Agency
CMS	Centers for Medicare and Medicaid Services
CNA	California Nurses Association
COBRA	Consolidated Omnibus Budget Conciliation Act
CPI	Consumer Price Index
DRG	Diagnostic Related Group
EPO	Exclusive Provider Organization

FAH	Federation of American Hospitals
FICA	Federal Insurance Coverage Act
FQHC	Federally Qualified Health Center
FTC	Federal Trade Commission
GAO	Government Accountability Office
GDP	Gross Domestic Product
HCPCS	Healthcare Common Procedure coding System
HHS	Health and Human Services, Department of
HMO	Health Maintenance Organization
HQA	Hospital Quality Alliance
HRSA	Health Resources and Service Administration
HSA	Health Savings Account
ICD-code	International Statistical Classification of Diseases Code
IOM	Institute of Medicine
IPAB	Independent Payment Advisory Board
JCAHO	Joint Commission on Accreditation of Healthcare Organizations
JCT	Joint Commission on Taxation
LPN	Licensed Practical Nurse
MAC	Medicare Administrative Contractor
MPFS	Medicare Physician Fee Schedule
NCQA	National Committee for Quality Assurance
NNA	National Nurses Association
NQS	National Quality Strategy
NSC	National Service Corporation
OECD	Organisation for Economic Co-operation and Development
PCORI	Patient-Centered Outcome Research Institute
PPHF	Prevention and Public Health Fund
PPO	Preferred Provider Organization

PRO   Peer Review Organization

PSO   Point of Service Organization

RBRVS   Resource-Based Relative Value Scale

SHOP   Small Business Options Plan

TANF   Temporary Assistance to Needy Families

VA   U.S. Department of Veterans Affairs

PREFACE

Each of the previous editions of this book outlined what the U.S. health care system looked like at the time. This edition directs attention to what the health care system looks like as of 2015. In reviewing what changed since the first edition, we can see a rising level of public dissatisfaction with our health care arrangements playing an increasingly important role. In the third edition, I discuss this and other factors that led to the epic health care reform plan, the Affordable Care Act (ACA) or Obamacare. In this the fourth edition, I examine the impact the law has had on the U.S. health care system since it was enacted in 2010. Discussion focuses on the ups and downs associated with the implementation process. I offer an assessment of the extent to which the law is or is not achieving the goals it set forth. In order to do that, I review efforts to identify appropriate indicators needed to gauge the law's impact.

I discuss mandates imposed by the law that have attracted the most attention. I also document changes that are being introduced without much public awareness. I identify the requirements affecting providers of health care goods and services that are actively reshaping the health care system.

The main message I wish to convey in this book is that the more one delves into the question of how our health care system is changing, the less certain we can be about whether what we have before us is working as well as we would like. In my view, neither castigating nor defending these arrangements is enough. Too many people are making suggestions about the health care system based on heartfelt beliefs or political opportunism. Making a cogent assessment of the strengths and weaknesses of our system and advocating change requires a good grasp on a lot of facts. The primary purpose of this book is to lay out those facts.

This edition of the book differs from previous editions in a number of ways. Most chapters end with questions related to the material presented in that chapter. I also suggest taking one or two quizzes that appear in the middle of serious discussions, quizzes authored by highly respected research organizations. And, I refer to some other media offerings, some less serious than others. In short, you can expect to encounter unexpected distractions in the midst of a lot of facts, figures, and mind-bending questions.

Many people have helped me construct the contents of this book. I am grateful to colleagues, especially those who have adopted previous editions, for the valuable feedback they have provided. Students' reactions have been important too because they have been good at catching me making assumptions about what I thought everybody already knew. As the references in the text indicate, I am indebted to an ever increasing number of dedicated researchers whose work I build on.

Sarah Stanton, senior acquisitions editor at Rowman & Littlefield, deserves special accolades for her continuing support and practical advice. Sarah's associates have been very helpful and patient in taking on the task of transforming messy manuscripts into polished books. Finally, I wish to acknowledge my husband's good nature in being willing to read multiple versions of early drafts and kindly explaining that the drafts could use clarification.

I

THE HEALTH CARE SYSTEM

An Overview

This book is about the U.S. health care delivery system. Its basic purpose is to explain how the health care system came to look the way it does. Special attention is devoted to examining how it is changing in response to the major health care reform legislation enacted in 2010, the Patient Protection and Affordable Care Act. The law has come to be known as the Affordable Care Act (ACA) or "Obamacare," a label President Barack Obama started using, largely robbing it of what was meant to be a negative connotation.

Americans have been expressing a good deal of disagreement about whether passage of the ACA should be celebrated, damned, or something in between. The calamitous "rollout" in the autumn of 2013, the first year that Americans were required to enroll in an insurance plan using newly created state Health Insurance Exchanges, confirmed the view on the part of some that the ACA was a disaster. Health Exchange Internet sites were unable to handle the huge number of inquiries. They crashed. The second enrollment period went well, so the calamitous rollout became old news. That does not mean that heated debates about the health care law went away or will be going away any time soon. Opinion polls continue to show that a significant proportion of people in this country are unhappy with the law. That and the fact that Republicans gained control of Congress in 2014 promising to repeal

Obamacare ensures that the ACA will be hitting the headlines again and again.

A short introduction to what the ACA was designed to achieve may be in order at this point. We will be discussing it in much more detail in later chapters. The primary objective of the legislation was to extend health insurance to as many people as possible, ideally achieving something close to "universal coverage." The law required everyone in the country to enroll in an insurance plan. Those who could not afford to do so would now qualify for a government-sponsored plan or receive a subsidy enabling them to enroll in a private plan. Large corporations were already insuring people although they were not obligated to do so by law. The ACA changed that. It requires all employers, except for the smallest ones, to insure their employees. The law instituted penalties to be imposed on both individuals and employers for noncompliance. Government-run insurance plans underwent considerable revision as well. The law also introduced measures aimed at improving quality of care and control over rising health care costs.

Whether or when Americans will change their minds about our health care system in general and the ACA in particular or agree on needed modifications in the law is hard to predict. What is your opinion at this point—should Congress get together with the president and fix what is wrong with the ACA? Or, should the plan be dumped? Then what, go back to the way things were? Start over and develop a new and better plan? These are obviously tough questions. In a moment you can see what other people say when asked a similar question.

IT'S STILL THE BEST HEALTH CARE SYSTEM IN THE WORLD

Americans have been registering a long list of things they don't like about our health care arrangements for quite some time. Yet the same Americans have also been likely to conclude that, in spite of all that, ours is still the best system in the world. Is it the best? Consider the most basic indicators, starting with life expectancy. Americans don't live as long as people in many other economically advanced countries. This is according to the U.S. Central Intelligence Agency (CIA) which, as you know, engages in spying on other countries in order to protect and promote U.S. interests. It also tracks life expectancy for 223 countries. The 2014 estimates indicate that life expectancy in the United States was 79.56 years.[1] If you think this is pretty good, consider the age attained by people in some other countries: Monaco, 89.57; Macau, 84.48. Granted, we don't compare ourselves with people in those countries. But Japan is third on the list at 84.46 and we do compare ourselves with the Japanese. Where does the United States stand? It appears that we are forty-second on the list. The CIA, as do most health care system analysts, considers infant mortality to be the most accurate indicator of a country's health status. The United States is fifty-fifth out of 224 on that list. That sure throws cold water on the idea that our system is the best.

As an aside I would like to make the point that there are those who respond to this kind of information by saying that negative information about the United States is put out by people intent on trashing this country. They can hardly say that about the CIA.

So what else do you hear people say makes our system the "best"? It's our technology, right? We have the best medical technology in the world, and we have lots of it. So why is it that all that technology is not succeeding in extending our life expectancy beyond that of so many other countries? Because people smoke, drink, eat the wrong things, don't exercise? Anyone who travels to other countries can't help but notice that people in many other countries smoke a lot more, drink more, eat rich foods, don't exercise, and still live a lot longer.

Finally comes the observation that so many foreigners come here to get health care services. Doesn't that prove that ours is the best health system in the world? My answer is that all those foreigners come here to get around what the Brits like to call the "queue," that is, the waiting line. In most countries, doctors decide whose case is most urgent and must be dealt with first. In this country, getting ahead of the line is a lot easier. Individuals, including foreigners, can and do get the services they want when they want them, if they are willing to pay for that privilege. Of course, this does sometimes have the effect of pushing Americans to the end of the line or out of the line entirely.

When pressed, the defenders of our health care system reluctantly acknowledge that some Americans may not benefit from what our system has to offer. Not because it isn't there, they point out, but because people aren't taking advantage of what is readily available. The defenders of our arrangements generally go on to say that highly sophisticated health care services and technology are available to everyone. Public hospitals and clinics have it and will provide it for free to those who can't pay for it. If people don't use it, you can't do anything to make them use it, that we are doing enough, and may, in fact, be doing too much. In my view folks not closely involved in studying the health care system and its impact on people in this country say this. They generally have little idea where free clinics can be found, how many there are, what kinds of services they provide, and so on.

If so many Americans think this is the best system in the world, how is it that Americans can also express a great deal of dissatisfaction about it? The contradiction becomes more glaring when we compare our answers to those of people in a number of other countries often mentioned in discussions about how ours should be changed. Table 1.1 is based on a 2013 study conducted by researchers associated with the Commonwealth Fund.[2] They surveyed people in fourteen economically advanced countries. (This list includes countries that we will be discussing in later chapters. We will also consider Japanese health care arrangements. Unfortunately Japan was not included in the study.) Respondents were asked: Which option would you choose in evaluating your health care system? a) the system works well, minor changes needed, b) fundamental changes needed, and c) needs to be completely rebuilt.

In assessing the results, the most striking observation is, of course, that more people in the United States say that they want the system rebuilt. But we should not overlook the fact that people in every one of these countries think their health care systems can be improved. It is just that far fewer of them think their systems should be totally rebuilt.

Table 1.1.   How Well the Health System Works

Country	Works Well	Fundamental Change	Rebuilt
Canada	38	51	10
France	42	47	11
Germany	38	48	14
Switzerland	46	44	8
UK	62	34	3
United States	29	41	27

The results of this survey add to the idea that the United States ends up looking like an outlier no matter what health care system indicator we look at, starting with life expectancy.

All one can say to sum up public attitudes regarding our health care system—saying our health arrangements are the best in the world and at the same time saying the system is so bad that it needs to be completely rebuilt—is that human beings have a unique capacity to hold two contradictory ideas in their minds at the same time.

BUT IT COSTS TOO MUCH

Then there is the matter of how much we pay for all this. Now this is something that Americans can agree on—that we pay way too much. However, exactly what it is that costs so much is not exactly clear. The cost of a doctor's visit? The drugs and tests that went along with the visit? The health insurance premium? The copay for the visit? All of these?

Health policy analysts interpret our complaints about how much it costs to mean that Americans are unhappy about how much they spend "out-of-pocket." Policy analysts are generally less concerned about that than how much the country as a whole is spending. So how much are we spending and how serious a problem is that? Let's look at CIA data on national health expenditures.[3] This time we are very near the top of the list. According to the CIA, we were spending 17.9 percent of our gross domestic product (GDP) on health care in 2011. (The most recent figure used by the Department of Health and Human Services is 17.4%.) The only countries that were spending more than we were at that time were Liberia at 19.50 and Sierra Leone at 18.80 percent, respectively. If mention of these countries rings a bell, it is because they were reporting the highest rates of mortality from Ebola in the autumn of 2014. If nothing else, these statistics tell us that spending such a large proportion of a country's funds on health care is no guarantee of good health. But let's take a closer look at what we are talking about when we discuss GDP.

The 17.9 percent figure that the United States spends might not sound so large until you consider everything else that falls under the GDP umbrella. The figure becomes more daunting if you conceptualize

GDP as a pie chart and understand that all goods and services produced or purchased by anyone and everyone in this country must fit into that pie chart—cell phones, cars, bridges, food, football game tickets, police protection, research on drugs to fight infectious diseases, rock concerts, social security payments, the wars in the Middle East, the space program. You get the picture. The health care slice of the pie has been getting bigger over the years. That means that the slices going to other categories have had to get smaller. Given that the health care share of the pie has gotten so big, whose slices are you willing to see get smaller?

Getting back to Liberia and Sierra Leone, the percentage of GDP they devote to health translated into dollars is small. That is because their total GDP, compared to that of economically advanced countries that produce and purchase enormous amounts of goods and services, is small. The CIA uses "purchasing power in the international marketplace" to estimate GDP. The numbers for 2013 are: Liberia $1,977 billion; Sierra Leone, $4,607 billion; and, United States, $16.72 trillion. It may be hard to get your mind around these numbers, but as you can see, the differences are gigantic. The fact that poor countries are spending a greater share of their GDP on health care leaves a lot less for everything else, making advancing the countries' economies an overwhelming challenge. No one is advising them to spend less on health care.

HEALTH SYSTEM GOALS

It is interesting to note that the public assessment of our health care system with regard to what makes our system great and how much it costs actually comes close to what health policy makers identify as health system goals. The goals are not formally documented and written down anywhere for good reason: we don't have an organized "system." Policy makers agree that any changes to our health care arrangements must focus on 1) *access*, 2) *quality*, and 3) *cost containment*.

Great goals, right? Unfortunately, this is where things get a little tricky. In part, because some analysts believe that you can only achieve any two out of three of the goals at any one time. Making things even more complicated is the fact that these objectives are impossible to define concretely and even more difficult to measure. What does "quality" mean? Who should define it?—doctors, patients, or some group of experts authorized (by whom?) to monitor quality? How much "access"? Does access mean that patients are entitled to have all the health care services they want? Or that they can pay for? Or that someone else, say, politicians, decides that they need? How do we measure "cost containment"? Do we want costs to drop or just not go up so fast? Are we prepared to cut anything the health system provides? Those are exactly the kinds of questions we will be addressing in the chapters that follow.

ANALYTICAL PERSPECTIVES

The fact that the public is not quite sure about the definitions of access, quality, and cost containment and how they should be tracked has not discouraged policy makers from attempting to come up with definitions and measures. What is special about this field of study is that scholars from multiple disciplines have been attracted to the field and have been struggling with these challenges. Not only has the study of health care systems evolved into an interdisciplinary enterprise, it has become an international, interdisciplinary enterprise. Scholars are interested in identifying the factors that explain enormous variations in mortality and morbidity that exist within countries and between countries. How much does access to health care services explain? How much of a role do other factors play, such as diet, education, genetics, and so on?

It is easy to understand why the field became both interdisciplinary and international once you consider the impact of the Internet. So much more information is accessible now than was true even a couple of decades ago. Information and interpretation of that information is being disseminated both more widely and more quickly. While this was happening, some other important developments were taking shape that would add even more information and an even wider scope of interpretation.

New nonprofit foundations focusing on health care and other related social trends started to appear and older, well-established foundations began to expand. Their intent was to speak to the educated public and to provide policy makers with relevant facts about issues on which the foundations wanted to take a stand. They hired researchers coming from various backgrounds who were charged with developing policy statements in language that the public would understand. We will be referring to reports issued by such organizations throughout the book.

Researchers working for government agencies began issuing reports as well. While data collected by the government has always been accessible to anyone who was interested, the files containing statistics presented in full are difficult to slog through. The fact that researchers on the inside of the data collection process were willing to present analyses of portions of that data in a timely manner was a welcome development. A number of new interdisciplinary academic journals leaning toward policy research have come into existence to make publication of all this new material possible. Again, expect to see references to these sources of data.

Material published by people in foundations and government agencies differs from work published by scholars in academic settings from which most of these researchers have come. In academia people from different disciplines had, and generally continue to have, no reason to work across disciplinary lines. In these new settings, highly trained researchers were suddenly forced to communicate with people who did not share the same disciplinary background and do so in a way that did not depend on the venerated academic tradition that requires discussion to be grounded in theory, typically theory exclusive to a particular discipline. This is to our advantage. People trained as physicians, public health researchers, epidemiologists, sociologists, economists, and political scientists, to name a few of the disciplinary backgrounds involved, are talking to each other and reading each other's work and working to make it comprehensible to the rest of us. However, you can still expect to encounter a lot of complex material, unfamiliar terms, and statistics.

BUILDING A SOCIAL INSTITUTION

Let's reflect on what people mean when they talk about the U.S. health care system. They are talking about a "social institution" that is the product of human effort. It is a structure that people are continually trying to reorganize largely because the process through which it was built has not been particularly neat and orderly. We know that the process is not about to stop in the case of the health care system, because so many observers continue to say that this system that we have collectively created is poorly organized, convoluted, and difficult to understand, not to mention far too expensive. People say many of the same things about other social institutions as well.

Those who study social institutions have in mind the processes and structures that exist to address a particular social need. The term "social institution" is not to be confused with the term "institution." We may refer to particular organizations, such as the Mayo Clinic, the Harvard Medical School, the Los Angeles County Hospital, as institutions because they are so old, well known, and widely respected. When scholars use the term "social institution," they are referring to all the organizations with connections to that particular sector of society—in this case the health care system. Yes, that makes it somewhat confusing. But we had to find a way to refer to multiple organizations operating in connection with each other. "Social institution" is the label we came up with. I offer this term as an example of a concept that scholars coming from other disciplines have adopted in talking about the health care system.

Health care arrangements were not considered from this perspective years ago when they did not attract nearly as much attention as they are attracting now. However, the health care delivery system has much in common with other social institutions, including education, religion, family, economy, and government. Like the other social institutions, it evolved to address a fundamental social need and was built on the same foundation as the others. Our basic cultural values, beliefs, traditions, and expectations about the behavior of others are the building blocks that serve as the foundation on which all social institutions are constructed. This explains why social institutions are so different from one society to another. Each society selects from its own stock of distinctive building blocks. I will continue to use the building blocks idea in referring to social values and expectations in other sections of this discussion.

True, most people have little to say about what social institutions look like. However, the choices made and opinions expressed by individuals and groups across the country are ultimately responsible for the ongoing process of shaping all of our institutions. There is generally no regularly scheduled opportunity to evaluate and possibly alter how social institutions operate. That is why we are devoting a fair amount of attention to public opinion surveys. The exception to this generalization is the political system. It functions with a schedule for voting on the persons and political parties who will govern for a set period of time.

The thinking regarding the operations of many other social institutions, including education, family, religion, and the economy, is harder to capture and document, which makes implementing society's preferences highly uncertain.

The social institution of education provides a good illustration. As I am sure you will agree, public schools receive a fair share of steady criticism, which periodically erupts into more aggressive demands for reform. There is always someone arguing that the schools are failing our children and proposing some way to remedy the situation—creating charter schools, relying more heavily on test scores to determine which schools to support and which to close down, getting rid of teachers whose students do not show improved test scores from one year to the next, and so on.

Another example of the scrutiny that social institutions undergo can be seen in the growing number of commentators who have been expressing alarm about the shifting role of religion in society. They say that we should be concerned about the steady drop in membership among traditional religions and the increase among fundamentalist sects. They argue that this brings with it more conservative views, a declining level of tolerance for behaviors such groups disapprove of, and a growing demand for restricting those behaviors. The battle over how to present sex education in schools, if at all, continues to attract the attention of parents, clerics, and other assorted interested parties. In such cases, we can also see two or three social institutions competing to establish control over the schools and schooling. Because it is not clear whose authority and preferences should come first, or if the problems they identify really require major changes, the debates and battles continue until enough people in society are prepared to either take sides or stop listening.

Then there is the family. People are not rushing to get married at an early age. People live together, some with the expectation of marriage in the future, some with no expectation of marriage. Marriage between same sex couples became legal in state after state over the last ten years. That is an exceptionally fast rate of change. Family as a social institution has obviously undergone a monumental transformation in a relatively short period of time. None of this was imposed on the citizenry. There was no systematic plan. Americans simply chose to change the structure of the family in light of shifting social values.

THE ORGANIZATION OF THE MATERIAL TO COME

There are a couple of things that I'd like to warn you about before we jump into this venture. First, as you become more involved in this discussion—and I do, of course, hope you will become very much involved—you will undoubtedly develop opinions about how you would like to see the system work. That's good! When you present your ideas to others keep in mind that your argument will be far more convincing if you can say why you are taking the position you are taking. In other words, try to refrain from sounding like you are preaching. As in: people *should* take better care of themselves, or there *should* be more health education, or the government *should* do this or that. Telling someone what they should do works best when it is accompanied by incentives, both positive and negative, what we often refer to as carrots and sticks. We all learned how that works at an early age—when Mom told us to put away our toys. Why would you do that if you liked to have the toys nearby whenever you wanted them? You were probably more willing to go along if Mommy said you could not go out and play with your friends if you did not pick them up. Or if Mommy said that she would take you to the new jungle gym just built in the community, but only if you picked up your toys. As such experiences made clear, it is easy to ignore what someone says you should do if there are no consequences, no accompanying rewards or penalties. In the case of arguing for health policy changes, you will be better off developing a strong argument regarding the impact of potential policy changes based on established facts as opposed to admonitions, making very clear the reasons people *should* be taking your recommendations seriously.

I suggest that you treat the statements made by policy makers similarly. If they cannot offer evidence based on a record of successes and failures of particular approaches to the problems they are discussing based on past experience, I would look at their recommendations with suspicion. The same holds true for critics who tell you what will happen if particular policies are enacted. It is easy to say what will happen if you don't have to bother with evidence.

Another point of discussion that deserves greater scrutiny is use of the term "socialized medicine." If one is referring to the systems that existed in Eastern European countries formerly affiliated with the Soviet Union, then talking about socialized medicine makes sense. The concept is also correct when applied to the system that exists in the United Kingdom, but generally not applied. When people use the term, they do so in order to argue that whatever they are objecting to is foreign and objectionable.

To say that something is socialized means that the government not only *runs* whatever it is, but *owns* all of the capital involved, and *employs* all of the personnel. Translating that into health care delivery system terms means the government has total control over all the resources—it owns all the buildings (hospitals, doctors' offices, clinics); hires, fires, and pays all the personnel (doctors, nurses, technicians, aides); and administers every step of the process (sets the budget, determines how many people to hire, what services to provide, where the offices should be located). This accurately describes the National Health Service in the United Kingdom. Other countries have a national insurance system. That is very different.

Countries that have "national health insurance" systems do not own hospitals or offices, and they do not pay the salaries of all health care personnel. Doctors who work in such countries may be paid directly by the patients who are then reimbursed by the national health insurance system or the doctors may simply bill the national health insurance system. With few exceptions, such as the Veterans Administration (VA) and some specially designated clinics, doctors in this country are paid this way. Other health care personnel are generally salaried by hospitals or other health care organizations. Hospitals in this country receive most of their income from the reimbursements that come through private insurance companies. In short, health insurance, whether it is a government plan or privately purchased plan, is nothing more than "an insurance plan." It works very much like car insurance.

As an aside, long waiting times for an appointment at the VA hit the news last year. Critics of government programs were quick to say that the VA was inefficient and incompetent. Some advocated an FBI investigation to identify fraud. When Congress looked into the matter, it became clear that the number of veterans had increased tremendously due to the wars in the Middle East but the VA budget had not increased. The VA simply did not have the funds to hire enough doctors. Congress increased the VA budget without further comment on inefficiency.

To sum up, I would like to say that this book is dedicated to the proposition that a firm grasp of the reasons behind past successes and failures of health care system modifications is essential to ongoing efforts to reorganize it. The chapters that follow constitute an effort to lay the groundwork for that. The more people who can be counted among the interested and informed, the more people will be in a position to evaluate how proposed changes to our health care arrangements will affect us. This is important because coming to this discussion as it is undergoing tremendous change means that we can all expect to hear a steady stream of contradictory proclamations regarding the implications of the health care reform legislation being tossed around by people representing all kinds of interests.

Also true is the fact that the implementation process, as troublesome as it is turning out to be, is certain to have a profound effect on the extent to which the programs and entities created by the ACA achieve the objectives specified in the law. As you probably know, many of those in a position to implement the policies enacted by the law have made it clear that they will resist doing so. Others in similar positions are struggling to comply with all the rules and regulations.

Consider the complications. The document defining the rules and regulations mandated by the law ran about 2,400 pages. It was to be introduced in stages over the next few years, but initial deadlines and some interpretations changed since then. New agencies were created tasked with creating measures and collecting data using those measures. States were given major responsibility for implementing key portions of the law. They all developed distinctive patterns for doing so. There are significant differences in how the law was designed to apply to individuals of different ages, incomes, and employment statuses. Regulations that require employers to provide health insurance for their employees differ depending on size of the organizations. Reimbursement going to providers of health care services, doctors and hospitals, were revised. And that is just a sample of the changes the law has introduced.

Trying to understand it all is mind-boggling. I will try to cover the basics. In order to substantiate what I say, I will offer facts and figures recognizing that we are being presented with new information every day. Fortunately most of it consists of updates rather than reversals of material that already exists. There is no way to keep all of it in mind, so I will provide you with sources, that is, the names of the organizations and agencies that are issuing the reports. This too presents complications because so much information is presented on-line rather than in hard copy. While that makes it easily accessible, there is no guarantee that all the documents will continue to be posted. You may end up going to the agency or organization that authored the document and find updated documents. No one said this would be easy, and I have to admit that it is turning out to be more challenging than I anticipated. So I can appreciate how difficult a time you will have slogging through it. All I can say is—hang in there!

Chapter 2 presents a synopsis of earlier reform efforts, public opinion data, and an overview of the social, political, and economic conditions that led to passage of the Patient Protection and Affordable Care Act. Chapters 3 and 4 focus on central components of the health care system—hospitals and health care occupations, respectively. Chapters 5 and 6 explain how health insurance works—first private insurance and then public insurance. Chapter 7 is devoted to health care systems in other countries. Chapter 8 outlines what we know about the performance of the ACA to date and goes on to consider alternative health care arrangements. Chapter 9 ends the discussion by returning to questions identified but not explored in earlier chapters. Most chapters end with specific discussion questions related to material presented in those chapters. As you will see, the discussion raises many questions. But as you will also see, coming up with answers is demanding and, in some cases, not necessarily conclusive.

2

OPINIONS ON HEALTH CARE REFORM

This chapter begins with a brief look at public opinion polls on the ACA and a number of other issues. The discussion goes on to consider previous health reform efforts, why they failed, and why health reform legislation finally passed in 2010. The chapter ends by outlining the policy alternatives from which the framers of the ACA had to choose in drawing up the legislation.

Let's stop for a moment and consider—is it possible that all the complaints that we have been hearing for such a long time about problems about our health system are just a matter of media hype and that things really aren't so bad? Yes, we all know that it is too expensive. However, as we noted in the last chapter, many Americans, even those who are not benefiting from it, are ready to say that ours is a great system. As we also know, there are very vocal critics out there who say that Obamacare is what is wrong with our health care arrangements. They say that it is a gross failure. We have all been exposed to heart-rending stories about individuals who had trouble with the health insurance exchange in their state, had their insurance dropped and now have to pay more, all accompanied by commentary on how this is all due to Obamacare and clearly shows that it is ruining America. Individual disaster stories about health insurance and a whole range of other topics would not be so common if media watchers had not established that the stories attract large enough numbers of viewers to convince sponsors to pay for advertising space. There are also stories about people who say that they would be having devastating health problems if not for Obamacare. However, you have to admit that a story about an individual, even a couple of individuals, tells us a lot about those cases and no more. Getting accurate information about how the ACA has affected large numbers of Americans requires a different approach.

It is also true that reports documenting the steady increase in the number of people who are newly insured, which are accompanied by graphs and statistics, keep coming out as well. Of course, they are not nearly as attention grabbing as stories about individuals and their troubles. There is no shortage of interested parties and political entities with a stake in how the ACA is perceived, so versions of both kinds of reports will continue to appear.

PUBLIC OPINION POLLS AND WHAT THEY TELL US

The media does pay a good deal of attention to the results of opinion surveys conducted by well-established polling organizations. The Henry Kaiser Family Foundation has been following public opinion and presenting its findings nearly every month since the ACA legislation was passed. Kaiser (for short) reports the results using a number of demographic variables including age, gender, race, income, and political affiliation. This is the question asked every month since the ACA was enacted:

> As you may know, a health reform bill was signed into law in 2010.
> Given what you know about the health care reform law, do you have
> a generally favorable or generally unfavorable opinion of it?

Remarkably, public opinion has remained stable. Near the end of 2014, 46 percent of the respondents said they have an unfavorable view; 41 percent a favorable view; others said they don't know or refused to answer.[1] It is worth noting that when specific parts of the law are explained to the respondents, the percentage of favorable responses increases significantly.

The authors of the Kaiser survey cannot control for how much respondents who are ready to register their opinion actually know about the law. While establishing how well informed respondents are about the law as a whole is not so easy, Kaiser has surveyed people to check their understanding of specific concepts that apply to the law. The analysis reveals considerable variation.

As an aside, you might consider taking the short quiz presented at the end of the Kaiser report. It could help prepare you for the material you will confront in chapters 5 and 6 when we get to how health insurance works in this country. The quiz is titled "Americans' Familiarity with Health Insurance."[2]

Then there is the survey conducted by that eminent pollster, Jimmy Kimmel. Yes, the comedian. The video of the on-the-street survey he conducted tells us a great deal about how informed Americans are about health care policy.[3] This is not exactly what you would call a scholarly piece of work, but it clearly exposes the fact that Americans are ready to register their opinion about the health care law regardless of how well informed they are. The fact that he is an entertainer and is going for laughs is apparent. But the fact that he chose to do this in front of a national audience does show that public opinion surveys have wide appeal, doesn't it?

Returning to the monthly polls carried out by the Kaiser Family Foundation, closer examination of the results tells us quite a bit more about who is registering positive or negative evaluations of the law. Asking the political affiliation of the respondents provides us with a graphic illustration of the political divide in the country. The question that asks respondents how favorably disposed to the law they are gives them four options to choose from: 1) expand what the law does, 2) move forward with implementing the law as it is, 3) scale back what the law does, or 4) repeal the entire law. Results are shown in table 2.1.

Sounds like the question we started with in the first chapter. It is interesting to see how differently people respond depending on their political affiliations, don't you think? But there may be more to the story on the split by political party than lack of understanding of the law. Consider the December 2009 CNN survey results on what people

Table 2.1.   Public Opinion Prior to Passage of the ACA (percent)

	Expand	Move Forward	Scale Back	Repeal
Democrats	34	40	8	8
Independents	20	16	20	29
Republicans	10	5	24	52

thought of the health care reform proposal prior to passage of the ACA.[4]

42 percent in favor
39 percent opposed because they thought it was too liberal
13 percent opposed because they thought it was not liberal enough
6 percent other and no opinion

It is apparent that some of those who were opposed to the health care reform legislation thought it was not liberal enough. In the end, the ACA did pass with a final vote in the House of Representatives of 291 to 212 without a single vote in favor by a Republican and with 34 negative Democratic votes. The Senate had to engage in some procedural maneuvering to get enough votes for passage. One of the stumbling blocks was resolved when coverage for abortions was dropped from the plan.

If the Democratic/Republican split suggests to you that we should assume that political party is playing a bigger role in determining public opinion than careful examination of the substance of the law, you might conclude that it is a good thing that some people are declaring themselves independents. And that they will be thoughtful and rational in their decisions rather than just following the party line. However, political scientists warn us not to put much confidence in that interpretation.[5] Those who have examined the position that independents take on various political issues say that the stance that some, not all, independents take can be explained by the fact that they are even less informed than those who identify with one party or the other. Indeed, political scientists express a good deal of despondency about how poorly informed the majority of Americans are about the full range of issues they are asked about.

We might take some consolation if those who were less informed were also less likely to vote. There is no reason to pin our hopes on that possibility either. It turns out that those who have the most to lose— that is, the uninsured—are the ones who are less likely to vote. This had a significant impact on the outcome of the vote during the last couple of national elections. The fact that so many independents did vote and very few of the uninsured voted gave opponents of health care reform, that is, Republican Party candidates, particularly Tea Party candidates, an advantage in the midterm election that took place at the end of

2010.[6] This voting pattern was repeated during the 2014 midterm election, when only 36.3 percent of the voters participated. In an opinion piece on November 11, 2014, the *New York Times* editorial board stated that voter turnout was the lowest it has been in seventy-two years, which the board interpreted as follows: "The reasons are apathy, anger and frustration at the relentlessly negative tone of the campaigns."

WHERE PEOPLE SAY THEY GET INFORMATION

Where people say they got their information on the law helps to clarify things a bit—prior to passage of the ACA 68 percent of respondents said they were getting their information from family and friends, 63 percent also mentioned cable, and 55 percent mentioned broadcast news programs. Of those who got their news from FOX News, 78 percent were opposed to the law. Of those who watched CNN, 52 percent favored the law.[7]

That the source of information is a major factor in whether Americans end up having a more favorable or less favorable stance toward the law is confirmed by the fact that one-third of seniors responding to the poll were convinced that the government was creating "death panels" that would be making end-of-life care decisions. Those who were getting their information from FOX News were more likely to register opposition on this basis than those getting their information from CNN.

The fact that Americans are unhappy about what has been going on in Washington, whether that has to do with the ACA or other legislation, is graphically illustrated by polls asking people how much confidence they have in the country's social institutions. The polls conducted by most major polling organizations reveal similar findings. The 2014 results of a poll conducted by Gallup asking Americans to indicate how much confidence they have in various social institutions may surprise you. Those being polled were presented with four options to express their assessments: "a great deal of confidence," "quite a lot," "some," or "very little." How much confidence they say they have in the three branches of government combines the "a great deal" or "quite a lot" answers; 30 percent expressed this level of confidence in the U.S. Supreme Court, 29 percent in the presidency, and 7 percent in Congress.[8]

The results are even more distressing when we look at the percentage who registered "a great deal of confidence" at 14 percent for the presidency, 12 percent for the Supreme Court, and 4 percent for Congress. According to Gallup, confidence in all three branches of government has reached a new low. Respondents were also asked how much confidence they have in news outlets; 12 percent reported having "a great deal of confidence" in newspapers, 10 percent in television news, and 8 percent for news on the Internet. Yet this is where people say they seek information on the health care system. Where else would most people look for information?

The National Opinion Research Center (NORC) at the University of Chicago, which has confidence data on thirteen social institutions going back to 1973, tells us that confidence in the Supreme Court has dropped down further than it has for the news media and the other two branches of government. The lack of confidence in government institutions and the media registered by the American public is much greater than it is for some of the other social institutions in the NORC poll, including the military, education, major companies, banks, and organized religion.[9] It is also worth noting that when NORC averaged out ratings over the 1973–2006 span for all thirteen of the social institutions it tracks, confidence in medicine came out at the top at 47.8 percent, followed by confidence in the scientific community at 40.3 percent.

HEALTH CARE REFORM: WHY NOW?

While there have always been a certain number of people in this country saying that we should be doing more for the underprivileged and underserved, many more people joined their ranks as indicators of the depth of the economic downturn that the country experienced during the first decade of the twenty-first century became more apparent. We experienced what has come to be known as the Great Recession which, according to the National Bureau of Economic Research, started in December 2007 and ended in June 2009. The recession was longer and more severe than any recession since the Great Depression of 1929. Many of the people who lost their jobs, their houses, and their savings did not recover and may never recover. They obviously don't think the recession ended in 2009, and they are not so sure that anyone is trying to help them. I mention this because it helps to explain what those people have to say about the direction in which this country is going.

A number of major developments have made it difficult for people to come to some consensus regarding government actions that might help the people hit hard by the recession. For example, there is the matter of the national debt. Whether the country should try to reduce the level of debt as fast as possible or take a little more time is a huge issue but one that many Americans apparently don't understand and others have strong views about, whether or not they understand the problem. From the perspective of some politicians, and some members of the public alike, attending to the national debt requires cutting back on government spending, including how much the government spends on health care. Others are opposed to the cutbacks because so many people would not be able to pay for health care.

The concern about being able to pay for health care as well as other goods and services is connected to something else that has been occurring in this country. The development that has been getting more attention over the last few years is the evidence indicating the steadily growing disparity between the rich and the poor. According to leading economists Thomas Piketty and Emmanuel Saez, economic inequality has not been this high since 1929. Saez reports that the income of those in the top 1 percent increased by 31.4 percent between 2009 and 2012. The income of those in the bottom 99 percent increased by 0.4 percent. [10]

A growing number of observers are saying that something must be done to reduce the level of socioeconomic inequality, which would, in turn, increase the pace of economic recovery while helping those hit by the recession. Yet arguing for government intervention flies in the face of what Americans are taught from an early age, namely that everyone in this country can succeed if they try. Indeed, some people are succeeding at unprecedented levels.

Consider executive pay. During the 1950s and 1960s, CEOs of major American companies took home about twenty-five to thirty times the wages of the typical worker. After the 1970s, the two pay scales diverged even more. In 1980, CEOs of big companies took home roughly forty times the average worker's wage; by 1990, one hundred times. [11] According to Elliot Blair Smith and Phil Juntz, writing for Bloomberg

Businessweek, the 2013 ratio was 495 times for the top 100 companies on its list.

The date at which this trend took off coincides with a number of other trends, most notably the growing split in social values. The 150th anniversary of the Civil War in 2011 gave scholars the opportunity to make some observations comparing that era to the current era. Some historians maintain that this country has not faced the degree of discord that we are facing now since the Civil War era. They note that religious fundamentalists opposed to social changes occurring then were responsible for divisiveness during the period leading up to the Civil War; and that it is religious fundamentalists opposed to social changes, particularly gay marriage and abortion rights, who are responsible for much of the divisiveness we are seeing now. For their part, the fundamentalists take the position that they cannot compromise on what they consider to be sin. Accordingly, they are willing to sacrifice a great deal, particularly economic benefits, to preserve principles that are central to their belief system.

The convergence of these two developments, a very high level of economic inequality and a very high level of divisiveness concerning social values, is causing schisms that are proving very difficult to overcome. The country's inability to come together to make changes in policies that govern our health system is grounded in these schisms as well.

It is important to recognize that this state of affairs actually serves the purposes of those who have reason to want to prevent social change. The message that those who are at the top of the economic ladder want to promote is that poor people have brought their problems on themselves—because they are lazy, have bad work habits, or indulge in other forms of personal waywardness, not because of the circumstances in which they find themselves. The people who are ready to accept this explanation for poverty are just as ready to claim that the reason some people have become very rich in the recent past is a combination of hard work and wise investment practices, and maybe one other critical factor: a healthy dose of good luck. The message is that the rich have achieved something that all Americans have a good chance of achieving. This helps to explain why so many Americans who are not at the top of the income ladder are opposed to social and economic change, even change that would benefit them. The unstated mantra is: don't change things before I get my chance!

At the same time, the media kept reporting that so many of the people who lost their jobs during the recession were, in fact, hardworking, upstanding members of our society who were committed to keeping their homes and way of life even as they were living from paycheck to paycheck—and that these were the folks who were now falling into poverty. While Americans may have been ready to acknowledge the truth of this observation, they were apparently not willing to think seriously about solutions to the problem and not especially interested in reflecting on how any of this affects the distribution of wealth.

Now that we have taken a closer look at the social environment that existed just prior to the passage of the health care reform law of 2010, let's look at society's response to the troubles people faced during the Great Recession of 2008 and compare that to society's response to the troubles people faced during the Great Depression of 1929. The Great Depression stands as a serious challenge to the idea that Americans will always take the position that individuals are at fault when they find themselves in financial difficulty. Americans seemed far more willing to accept the idea that good, hard-working people could suffer financial loss then, than they are now. Indeed, this insight was responsible for passage of the Social Security Act of 1935.

HOW SOCIAL SECURITY CAME TO BE AND THE FUNCTION IT SERVES NOW

We focus on the social security program in order to reflect on why it came into existence in the first place, and to understand the role social security plays now in validating eligibility for the receipt of government health care benefits among persons over sixty-five years of age.

The Social Security Act was passed in recognition of the plight of the elderly after the economic crash of 1929. Everyone understood that the elderly were far less likely to find employment in the wake of the Great Depression than were younger people. Remember, laws against age discrimination did not exist then, so people could be forcibly retired at age sixty-five. On the other hand, there is no evidence to suggest that the elderly were clamoring for this program. They were proud

Americans accustomed to solving their own problems with the help of family members. They were opposed to government assistance defined as welfare. In other words, they shared the cultural values of the society in which they were living.

Social security became acceptable to the elderly, as well as to other members of society, when it was presented as social insurance, that is, a pension that workers would earn by contributing through a payroll tax over their work lives. The payroll tax or Federal Insurance Coverage Act (FICA) tax would go into the Social Security Trust Fund and be available upon retirement to the individual at age sixty-five.

The FICA tax was designed to rise little by little. It stands at 6.2 percent as of 2015, with the employee paying 6.2 percent, and the employer paying 6.2 percent. Observers periodically raise concerns about the solvency of the trust fund. The problem on the horizon a few decades ago was that the baby boom generation would be reaching retirement age as of 2011. This was expected to create an imbalance between the number of people contributing to the fund and the number of people receiving benefits. The question of how to address this eventuality brought a wide range of commentators into the discussion. More recently, concern shifted to the impact of the economic downturn. Fewer people were working and contributing to the trust fund. In actuality, people over the age of sixty-five are continuing to contribute because many are not retiring, which is creating other problems such as the lack of jobs for younger people. But that is not a problem that we can address here.

Observers repeatedly mention the increase in life expectancy we have achieved since 1935 in discussing the solvency of the Social Security Trust Fund. After all, life expectancy in 1935 was fifty for men and sixty-two for women. Yes, these were indeed the official life expectancy figures at that time; however, it is important to understand that life expectancy is actually calculated based on the total mortality rate, including infant mortality. That complicates things because the first year of life is the most dangerous. Mortality during that year is especially high. According to the Social Security Administration, the more appropriate measure is *adult life expectancy*. When we look at that measure, we find that men who reached the age of sixty-five in 1940 could expect to live for another 12.7 years, and women could expect to live another 14.7 years. The most recent projections do show substantial gains in life expectancy. Males who reach age sixty-five currently can expect to live another 17.7 years, and females can expect to live another 20.3 years. So we really are living longer. However, understanding what life expectancy figures mean and how they are calculated makes the issue more complex, don't you think?

After deliberating the implications of increasing life expectancy for the Social Security Trust Fund in 1983, Congress instituted a new schedule for retirement, with full benefits incrementally increasing the age of eligibility from age sixty-five to age sixty-seven on a month-by-month basis. Americans have always been able to retire earlier, at age sixty-two, with reduced benefits. That has not changed.

The solvency of the trust fund was still not assured even after this adjustment. That led Congress to ask the trustees to assess the situation once again in 2008. This time the trustees indicated that the trust fund would be running out of money by 2017. The time estimate keeps getting revised, but the prediction that the fund will run out of money continues. The options in 2008 were to either reduce benefits or increase taxes or some mix of both. Some argued for privatization, which translates into giving people the pension they had accrued as a lump sum to be invested as they wish. Others advocated investing the trust fund in stocks, bonds, and other financial instruments, that is, in the market. The severity of the Great Recession dampened public enthusiasm for investing in the market. The topic continues to come up without a solution that the majority in Congress and the public sphere can agree on.

Curiously, the media has made little mention of the ceiling on FICA taxes in discussions about the solvency of the trust fund. In 2015, the FICA tax applies to income up to $118,500. The ceiling goes up a bit each year. However, income above that ceiling is *not taxed*. Economists point out that this is a "regressive" tax. In other words, it places a bigger burden on people at lower income levels and relieves people at higher income levels from having to pay any taxes on earnings over $118,500. That obviously limits the amount of money being contributed to the trust fund.

HEALTH CARE REFORM, 1935–1965

There was some effort to incorporate health care benefits when the Social Security Act was legislated, but coming out of the Depression, the country simply could not afford it. In fact, health care reform had been taking a backseat to other issues on the national agenda through-out the first half of the twentieth century for a long list of reasons. To begin with, medical costs were not very high and doctors were much more willing to accept token payment, a chicken or having some house repairs done, when patients could not afford to pay the fee.

Another reason why health care reform did not receive more atten-tion during this period is that, while the effects of the Great Depression lingered on during the decade of the 1930s, the country's attention turned to the demands brought on by World War II. Everything changed with the onset of the war. War production went into high gear. As more men became engaged in war activities, women entered the work force—working in offices and in factories. They saved the money they made, in part because consumer goods were not available since they were not being manufactured. When the war ended, Americans were eager to make up for lost time. They bought new houses in the suburbs and cars to get there. They bought new furniture and appli-ances for the new houses. They had babies—creating the baby boom generation. The economy was booming. Personal income increased by 37 percent between 1950 and 1956.[12]

Health care reform did come up for serious debate during the post-war period, the late 1940s, which was the Truman era. It is interesting to see what people thought about health reform then; 82 percent of the public favored doing something to help people pay for health care and that 68 percent agreed that using social security as the basis for enacting a universal health care plan was a good idea.[13] Despite this high level of popular support, the proposed plan did not succeed for complicated political reasons.

Health care reform did not capture the attention of the public again until the early 1960s. Interest in health care reform during this era was inspired by the observations offered by a few highly respected social critics who pointed out that not everyone in the country was enjoying the newfound postwar prosperity. While the critics presented powerful impressionistic information, there were no factual data to which anyone could refer in discussing the scope of the problem. The government was pressed into figuring out how many poor people there were and who they were. There was no standard indicator in existence at the time that would produce a count of the number of poor people in the country. The government first had to establish a measure to determine who was poor and who was not before doing a count. The Bureau of Labor Statistics was mandated to take on the task. It turned to the Consumer Price Index (CPI), which it had been using to set wages for workers in shipbuilding yards. The CPI involved calculation of the cost of a market basket of goods that a person would need to survive—starting with food, going on to clothing, housing, transportation, medical care, and a number of other categories, like energy.

The cost of a basket of essential goods and services, announced for the first time in 1961, was calculated to be $2,973 for a family of four. This established the *poverty line*. Those whose income was less than that were considered poor. So how many people were found to be poor and who were these people? More than one out of every five persons, 22 percent, turned out to have an income lower than the poverty line. Of persons between the ages of twenty-five and fifty-four, 13 percent were found to be poor; but, 47 percent of those over sixty-five were poor.[14] Of those in female-headed households 50 percent were poor; and 56 percent of African Americans were poor. The fact that this took place during the Kennedy/Johnson era, when the mood of the country was considerably more sympathetic to the plight of the needy than has been true since then, explains why the findings came to be defined as a serious national problem that the government needed to address.

The social values that prevailed during that period meant that Americans were more likely to be concerned about the plight of all the categories of people identified as poor. A range of social programs was legislated during this period designed to address problems faced by specific categories of people. Medicaid, civil rights legislation, and funding for education and training at all levels came into existence at this time. The fact that the elderly were having difficulty paying for health care even though they were receiving social security checks captured the attention of the country. The majority of Americans, 75 percent according to surveys conducted at the time, said they favored a plan to provide medical care for seniors.[15] This led to passage of the Medicare program in 1965.

However, policy experts did not anticipate that the costs of health care would continue to increase after the two massive government-sponsored health insurance programs, Medicare and Medicaid, came into existence. They projected a decline in health care costs once the needs of the underserved were addressed. What in retrospect looks like a relatively small but steady increase in health care costs led to the next significant piece of health care legislation. The Nixon administration introduced a major health care reform in 1974 designed to encourage people to seek care early before problems got more serious. Policy experts reasoned that providing preventive care and addressing health problems at an early stage when they were less costly to treat should stem the rise in health care costs. This accounts for the origins of Health Maintenance Organizations (HMOs), which we will discuss in more detail in chapter 5.

While the cost of care continued to rise, in fact, at a faster rate than it had been rising until then, health care reform received little attention during the 1980s. Americans had been hearing about the number of people who did not have health insurance and could not afford to obtain health care, but it was only when Bill Clinton entered the political arena during the late 1980s that doing something about the health care reform became a primary goal. In fact, health care reform became one of the basic elements in Clinton's political campaign. He came into office in 1990 with 66 percent of Americans saying they favored legislation creating a tax-funded national health insurance plan.[16] Pundits found many reasons to explain why the plan never made it to the proposal stage for Congress to consider.

One explanation is that corporate executives were convinced that the plan would not succeed so it made no sense to risk coming out in support of it. That would have displeased too many influential people associated with the business sector. Ironically, many companies, particularly in the auto industry, would have benefited tremendously from the passage of health care reform. It would have reduced operating costs and given manufacturers a significant pricing advantage in the international market. In short, political interests trumped economic interests.

Debates about health care reform continued to attract the public's attention over the next two decades because health care costs continued to rise and increasing numbers of people were having trouble getting health insurance. The economic downturn during the early years of the first decade of the twenty-first century exacerbated the problem because people were losing their health insurance along with their jobs. In other words, more people could not get health care services because they could not afford to pay for health care and they could not find health insurance coverage that would make health care affordable.

This is a good place to stop and see the extent to which poverty may have been a factor in people's inability to obtain health care and other goods and services over the last few decades. So how many people are we talking about? How many Americans are poor as of the second decade of the twenty-first century? What do poverty statistics look like after all those interventions aimed at reducing poverty over the last five decades? According to the Census Bureau, the poverty rate stands at 14.5 percent as of 2013. Statistics for specific categories of people, based on 2011 figures, were considerably higher for some categories: 27.2 percent in the case of African Americans and 25.6 percent of Hispanics, compared to the 9.7 percent rate for non-Hispanic whites and 11.7 percent rate for Asians.

A closer look at age and poverty suggests that we have not been attending to the emergence of a new poverty problem. The numbers have shifted from high numbers of poor elderly to high numbers of poor children. The 2012 count reveals that 21.3 percent of all children under age eighteen were poor; the rate fell to 19.9 percent as of 2013. Of children in a female household with no husband present, the rate was 47.2 percent. By contrast, less than 9.5 percent of persons over sixty-five fell below the poverty line in 2012, a figure that is lower than the poverty rate of those of working age between eighteen and sixty-four, 13.6 percent of whom are poor. So now that you have considered the face of poverty in this country, would you say that things have gotten better and that we are moving in the right direction to address poverty, and the problems associated with it like lack of health insurance, or would you say that we are not doing nearly enough? This is the question that will keep coming up from one chapter to the next.

FACTORS THAT EXPLAIN THE SUCCESS OF THE 2010 HEALTH CARE REFORM

Researchers who reviewed fifty opinion polls conducted since 1943 (twenty-three of those conducted between 2008 and 2010), have given us a far more detailed picture of the factors that kept health care reform from being legislated until 2010. It is interesting to see what has changed and what has stayed the same. It seems that Americans have consistently registered support for health care reform, but that their support has usually been tempered by overriding concern about the economy. Americans have consistently registered dislike for personal sacrifice; while they have favored reforms that would provide health insurance for the uninsured all along, they have not been interested in making personal sacrifices in order to pay for that. They are inconsistent now, just as they have been in the past, in saying that they like the health care arrangements they have on the one hand and saying they are worried about being able to pay for needed care on the other hand. This assessment is worth keeping in mind to see how our values compare to those of people in other countries, which we will address in chapter 7.

What changed to make passage of the ACA possible is that the framers of the law figured out how to meet a formidable challenge—altering the health care system without upsetting those who like their current arrangements. Shifts in attitude exhibited by major health sector players prior to passage of the ACA played a particularly noteworthy role. Insurance companies stopped running ads accusing government of taking over people's right to choose their own health care plans. They stopped saying that health care reform signaled a socialist takeover, which is not to say that others opposed to government programs and government spending stopped invoking the specter of government takeover. The professional associations representing hospitals, doctors, and nurses, each to a different extent, began saying that the country's health care system was broken and should be fixed. They differed in how they thought it should be fixed, but they were no longer putting up a wall against health care reform proposals. In other words, influential health sector participants began to see that they could benefit from reforms that would provide more people with health care coverage.[17]

Undoubtedly the most important factor responsible for passage of the ACA was the fact that Democrats were in control of all three government bodies involved in enacting laws in this country—the White House, the House of Representatives, and the Senate during the first two years of the Obama administration. The Democrats were the ones proposing health care reform each time it came up for serious discussion over the last century. This is the first time in a long time that they had the leverage and political savvy to make it happen.

However, things change. Given that the 2014 midterm election shifted control over Congress from the Democrats to the Republicans, would you say that this means that the public wants the ACA repealed, which is what leading Republicans have been promising? Or do you think that the *New York Times* editors, quoted earlier in this chapter, have it right in saying that the vote means that Americans are both apathetic and angry? Or that the country is unhappy with Washington and wants to see the two parties work together to make adjustments to the law so that it works better for people? We simply have to watch to see how the political wrangling plays out. It may not take very long either since campaigns for the next election now start even before the results for the current election are in. And the ACA promises to be one of the core issues under debate over the next few years, possibly for years after that.

HEALTH CARE REFORM OPTIONS

The crux of the matter in understanding why the ACA passed is recognizing how the framers of the ACA legislation succeeded in altering basic health care system arrangements without upsetting those who did not want their own arrangements changed. That can be explained by identifying the options for making changes they had to choose from. How they managed to juggle those choices is a testament to political shrewdness. According to the Institute of Medicine (IOM), based on the structure of previous health care reform proposals, the framers had four options to choose from to attain universal health insurance coverage, which the IOM was advocating.[18]

As an aside, the IOM's observations receive a great deal of attention due to its long-established history and the high level of respect it garners from all quarters. The IOM was established in 1970 as an arm of the National Academy of Sciences, which was chartered under President Abraham Lincoln in 1863. It issues reports based on the conclusions arrived at by the experts it brings together "to facilitate discussion, discovery, and critical cross-disciplinary thinking." It responds to requests from Congress, other agencies, and organizations. The experts who are invited to participate are reimbursed for expenses but receive no compensation.

The four options outlined by the IOM are as follows:

1. An *employer mandate* requiring employers to provide insurance for all employees and all others to be covered by public plans;
2. An *individual mandate* requiring everyone to buy their own insurance with the aid of tax credits;
3. An *incremental approach*, that is, expansion of existing public programs—Medicare, Medicaid, SCHIP (State Children's Health Insurance Program), often together with government assistance to allow the uninsured to buy into these programs;
4. The *single payer plan*.

For a long time, the third option was the only one most Americans would support. What makes the health care reform of 2010 so extraordinary is that it succeeded in rolling the first three alternatives into one proposal, leaving out only the fourth option, the single payer plan. It is the single-payer option that has consistently produced the strongest opposition because it is so dependent on government control over health insurance arrangements rather than competition among private insurance companies.

What was unique about the ACA is that it succeeded in bundling a liberal goal—health insurance coverage for everyone—together with a conservative approach to insurance, in other words, personal responsibility for selecting a health plan of one's own choosing. That allowed the individual mandate, requiring everyone to buy health insurance, to go forward. The employer mandate, which has most impact on small employers, could be included because the government would be providing tax relief for small employers in order to ease the financial burden. While the law does expand government programs, it leaves control over provision of health insurance in the hands of the private sector. This was the critical factor allowing passage of the ACA.

Policy makers responsible for the ACA left the fourth option on the table. But it has not gone away. We will discuss what proponents of this option have to say about it in chapter 8.

QUESTIONS AND ISSUES TO THINK ABOUT

You can expect to find questions at the end of most of the remaining chapters. The questions presented in this chapter are "thought" questions rather than "policy" questions.

- Children now constitute the largest category of poor persons in the country. They cannot do anything about their poverty. Nor can they get health insurance on their own. There are provisions for insuring poor children, but the processes vary from state to state, leaving many children uninsured. The first question is: Should we, as a society, do more to provide health insurance for children? If we agree that this is a problem that deserves our attention, the next question is: what is the best way to address the problem? Fix the current system? Come up with a more organized and targeted plan? What about children born here of parents who are not legal immigrants? What we have here is a mix of value judgments and practical solutions that cannot be separated. I raise these questions because they elicit views grounded in values. I do not suggest that you develop policies to address these questions before you know a lot more about existing health policy.
- Next, let's consider the problem that the confidence in social institutions surveys reveal. Clearly this is a problem that has gotten worse with no remedies in sight. But is a problem that is worth thinking about. There is also the problem of needing a source of information about the health care that everyone can trust. Got any ideas about how to deal with the problem of trust in social institutions and more specifically a place to turn to for information on health care?

3

HOSPITALS AND OTHER
HEALTH CARE ORGANIZATIONS

Why talk about hospitals? What's so interesting? People generally don't think about them unless they need to go to one because of a pressing health problem. When they do go, they are naturally preoccupied with the health problem that is causing them to be there. For purposes of this discussion we will be taking a broader view of hospitals. We will look at hospitals and other health care organizations as organizational structures, who owns them, how much we are spending on hospital care, and how hospitals and related organizations are changing. How much we are paying is an attention-getter. As of 2011, we were paying about $10,000 per hospital stay. Who can afford that? Then there is how much of the country's health care dollar was going to hospitals—about $387.3 billion.[1] Shouldn't we be asking—can we afford THAT? I don't propose to answer the question, but you have to admit that it is worth considering more closely to see why we are spending so much.

Before we get to that, let's look at a number of basic descriptive characteristics that distinguish hospitals from each other. The most basic difference stems from how long patients stay in the hospital. There are short-term stay, or "acute care," hospitals and there are long-term stay hospitals. The majority of hospitals in this country are short-stay hospitals. Long-term stay hospitals generally provide inpatient mental health treatment and rehabilitation. Also, some long-term care facilities are not hospitals, but nursing homes. Unless otherwise indicated, the discussion to follow refers to short-term, acute care hospitals.

Size is another meaningful characteristic. Counting the number of hospitals tells you something, but leaves a lot unsaid about capacity, that is, what services the hospitals are capable of delivering. There are various ways to measure capacity, including the hospital's number of employees, annual budget, kinds of specialty units, number of branches, and so on. The commonly agreed-on measure of size is the number of beds the hospital maintains. A hospital in a rural area might have 50 to 75 beds, although such small hospitals are disappearing, while a medical center hospital can have over 900 beds.

Another basic distinguishing criterion is hospital ownership. Who owns the hospital makes a significant difference; the extent of the difference has inspired heated debate over the past few decades. When the government reports hospital statistics, it differentiates between hospitals owned by the federal government and nonfederally owned hospitals. Federally owned and funded hospitals are basically operated by either the Veterans Administration (VA) for the exclusive use of veterans of the armed forces or military hospitals used by active members of the armed forces. All other hospitals fall into the nonfederal category. They are divided into three ownership categories: 1) nonprofit, 2) for-profit, and 3) state-local government.

Hospitals in the state and local government category are the easiest to recognize. They are usually named to clearly indicate that they are government-sponsored, like Boston City Hospital, Los Angeles County Hospital, or University of Illinois Hospital. The state and local government hospitals are, in the broadest sense, not-for-profit organizations. They are typically referred to as *public* hospitals, meaning that that they are supported by the public through state or local taxes.

Major university-sponsored teaching hospitals usually, but not always, carry the name of the university that administers the associated medical school. A recent trend is naming a university hospital building if not the whole hospital after a major donor. Medical schools have more graduates than they can accommodate at the university hospital for residency training, which takes anywhere from three to five years, more if the doctor wishes to subspecialize. For this reason, university teaching hospitals must develop ties to state and local as well as "community" hospitals to provide places for medical students and residents to receive hands-on training.

The term "community" hospital has traditionally served as a catchall label for hospitals that are owned and operated for the benefit of the community. They may have been established by religious orders, by leading citizens who aim to create a hospital to provide for their own religious or ethnic groups, or by residents of a particular geographic community. Such hospitals operate on a nonprofit basis. People employed by the hospital receive a salary but do not share in hospital profits and no investors share in profits. In reporting statistics, the government is now using the "community" label more broadly to refer to all acute-care hospitals not owned by the government.

For-profit hospitals are privately owned and operated as businesses, that is as profit-making organizations. They are not always easy to distinguish from nonprofit community hospitals. Historically for-profit hospitals were owned by individuals, usually one or more doctors. As owners, they pocketed what they earned from running the hospital; they made all the decisions on the need for improvements, both technological and cosmetic, hiring staff, and so on. They also paid taxes on any profits. This is a major distinction. The federal government does not tax nonprofit hospitals. In order to qualify for this designation, a hospital must develop a charitable care plan for providing care to a clearly identified category of persons. "Bad debt," the result of patients not having the money to pay for their care, is not the same thing as a plan. Hospitals may lose their nonprofit status if they do not come up with a plan.

Over time for-profit hospitals shifted from ownership by a few doctors to corporate ownership (to make things more confusing, corporations that sell stock are sometimes referred to as "publicly owned" because many people are owners by virtue of investing in the company). For-profit corporations are established by law to make a profit, sell shares, and distribute profits to stockholders who invest in the business.

The U.S. Department of Health and Human Services (HHS), which keeps track of the number of hospitals in each category, reports that the number of government hospitals has been declining and the number of for-profit hospitals has been increasing. The total number of hospital beds has also been declining, but the number of beds in for-profit hospitals has been increasing. Before we get to what accounts for these trends, let's go back to the beginning of the twentieth century to see how we got to the current number of hospitals and hospital beds.

A BRIEF HISTORY OF THE MODERN HOSPITAL

Before the twentieth century, people avoided a hospital stay if they had any choice about it. Hospitals were essentially charitable organizations that provided basic care and housing for indigents who had no place else to go. Exactly how many hospitals there were in this country around the turn of the century is difficult to determine. According to one of the few estimates available there were only 178 as of the mid-1880s.[2] People did not go into a hospital willingly because everyone knew that hospitals were dangerous places. One's chances of dying once you were in the hospital were high. Middle-class people certainly would not have paid to go there. Those who could afford it were treated in their own homes or the doctor's office. Many people also sought advice and remedies from the apothecary (i.e., pharmacist) and any number of other kinds of health practitioners.

While most people would have been reluctant to go into the hospital at the beginning of the twentieth century, surgeons were beginning to find it more difficult to perform surgery outside of the hospital. They had begun to perform more new kinds of surgery than they had been able to do even a few decades before largely due to a range of technological advances. Anesthesia, which was initially developed in the 1840s, had become more effective and reliable. (Imagine what surgery was like before anesthesia! People died from the shock of being cut open even before they had a chance to develop an infection; if they survived, infection was highly likely.) The value of antisepsis (a sterile surgical environment) was discovered in the 1860s and was now fully implemented. X-ray technology came into existence in the 1890s. As surgeons became more dependent on hospitals to perform surgical procedures, they also became more interested in setting standards that would improve the quality of hospital care.

Accordingly, in 1918 the American College of Surgeons (ACS) began inspecting hospitals in an effort to assure the public that hospitals were well equipped and that the doctors doing surgery were well qualified. They did so by encouraging doctors to assume greater responsibility for overseeing the work of their colleagues. They were especially concerned about preventing less qualified or unethical colleagues from performing unnecessary surgery. The medical profession as a whole, led by the most accomplished surgeons, improved the quality of care provided in hospitals by having pathologists perform autopsies on the patients who died in the hospital to determine whether the diagnosis was accurate and the surgery was truly necessary and, of course, done well. The public nature of the autopsy meant that surgeons had to be more careful about the surgeries they were performing, because all doctors affiliated with the hospital were encouraged to attend autopsies as an excellent method to discuss cases and advance medical knowledge. Having colleagues discover that the surgeon was misdiagnosing patients and performing unnecessary surgery would certainly not be good for the surgeon's reputation. (Autopsies have become too costly to perform on a routine basis. They are done at the request of parties willing to pay for them, namely families of the deceased and law enforcement agencies. They are also performed by medical residents for training purposes.)

To ensure that autopsies were, in fact, being carried out and that the privileges of doctors doing inappropriate surgeries were restricted, the ACS encouraged doctors to become active members of the medical staff organization in the hospital. In short, doctors were encouraged to establish firm control over the day-to-day work taking place in hospitals.

Getting back to the early years of the twentieth century, administrators of hospitals were well aware of the fact that their interests were not identical to those of surgeons, or for that matter, the interests of other physicians and other hospital personnel. They began organizing themselves into an association of their own. In 1899 they established the Association of Hospital Superintendents of the United States and Canada, which became the American Hospital Association (AHA) within the next few years. For-profit hospitals formed their own association in 1966, the Federation of American Hospitals (FAH), which identifies itself as the "national representative of investor-owned and managed community hospitals."

Over the next decade or so the AHA came around to the view of the surgeons that raising hospital standards was important and that inspections were essential. However, the AHA did not have the resources or the power over hospitals to impose such inspections. The ACS did have that power.

When hospitals were primarily charitable institutions, doctors contributed their services. They did so because hospitals provided them with interesting "clinical material" (i.e., interesting cases). In other words, the patients were more likely to be in an advanced stage of disease because they did not have the money to obtain treatment earlier, often because the disease prevented them from working and impoverished them. Many very sick people could not afford to see a doctor privately. So doctors volunteered their services in exchange for the opportunity to treat the interesting cases. As hospital care improved, middle-class patients began asking to be admitted to the hospital, indicating willingness to pay the doctor as well as the hospital for the care they would receive. Thus began a pattern that would lead to hospitals beginning to depend on paying patients for their operating funds. Surgeons were in a position to funnel their paying patients to the hospital of their choice. Hospitals were left with little alternative but to accede to the surgeons' wishes—focusing on making the improvements that surgeons demanded, such as bigger and better surgical suites, more advanced equipment, and more staff.

The American Hospital Association first approached the ACS around 1950 to explore the possibility of setting up a cooperative inspection program. Four organizations joined together to develop hospital accreditation standards: the American Hospital Association, the ACS, the American Medical Association (AMA), and the American College of Physicians (ACP). By 1952 they had worked out standards and established a new organization, the Joint Commission on Hospital Accreditation, to carry out the inspections. The inspections were to be voluntary; hospitals would have to request them and be charged for the costs of carrying them out. As of 1987, it became the Joint Commission on Accreditation of Healthcare Organizations (JCAHO), generally referred to as the Joint Commission. The role of the Joint Commission is obvious to everyone employed in a hospital, especially when the Joint Commission arrives for an accreditation visit. In response to critics who said that in preparing for the visit, hospitals could organize material so that errors would be less apparent, the Joint Commission has instituted unannounced visits.

Hospitals expanded rapidly during the first few decades of the twen-tieth century, until the end of the 1930s.[3] According to one of the first AMA counts, there were approximately 4,300 hospitals in the country in 1928. Then the trend suddenly reversed. The drop is attributed to the Great Depression. Patients could not afford to go to a hospital, those who were taken there because it was an emergency could not pay for it, and many smaller hospitals did not survive. The hospitals that did sur-vive could absorb such losses only because they were receiving support from especially dedicated and, in many cases, wealthy contributors. Some hospitals survived because of the support they received from religious orders or an entire ethnic community. The only other hospitals that survived the Depression were the public hospitals.

The hospital sector changed little between the Depression and the end of World War II. Once the war ended, however, the country expe-rienced a period of adjustment that brought with it not only peace, but a period of unprecedented prosperity and expansion into newly devel-oping communities. With all this expansion, there was a need for new hospitals, which brought the Hill-Burton Act into existence in 1946. The federal government matched the funds raised by the community for the purpose of building a new hospital or adding on to an existing one. Consequently, established hospitals expanded and new community hospitals sprang up all across the country.

Was there really a need for so much more hospital construction or could there have been some other reason behind the urge to build and expand? Admittedly, the definition of "need" in this case has its own body of literature. For purposes of this discussion, let's say that some-thing besides objective need is involved. Many hospitals came into exis-tence for symbolic reasons. They stood as a major source of pride to the community whether it was an ethnic, religious, or geographical commu-nity. The Hill-Burton Act provided the perfect opportunity to act on that sense of pride. It is also true that some urban hospitals were built by people who had good reason to believe that they were not welcome in hospitals operated by other groups. Jewish doctors, for example, ex-perienced discrimination when seeking privileges in hospitals run by others. Jewish patients felt better being treated by doctors who they felt would understand their cultural values. Similarly, Catholic hospitals of-fered the assurance that patients could practice their religion and that priests would be readily available to offer solace, hear confession, and offer last rites. Immigrants were concerned about being able to communicate and wanted to be able to speak their own language in the hospital. Finally, the newly established suburban communities were interested in proving that they could offer everything that the city could offer, only newer and better. (See the social construction of reality at work here? The people building hospitals were certain there was a need for all those new hospitals and new additions—perhaps not the kind of need that policy analysts might be looking for, but, as you can see, "need" is in the eyes of the beholder.) It goes without saying that poor people in poor neighborhoods could not, and did not, take advantage of the Hill-Burton funds. For this reason, new hospitals were not built in many communities that really needed them. Distribution of hospitals did not get better. As the initial benefactors moved out of some neighborhoods and other groups moved in, hospital support systems faltered and the hospitals closed down.

Aside from community pride, one other factor that played a major role in fostering hospital expansion coincidentally came into play just after World War II ended. Synthesized penicillin came into existence during the late 1940s and became widely available by 1950. The availability of penicillin had a major effect on hospital expansion because this was the first time that hospitals could control infection with certainty. Prior to that time drugs to control infection did exist, but none was as powerful as the new series of antibiotics, starting with penicillin.

But things change. We are now encountering "super bugs," such as Methicillin-resistant *Staphylococcus aureus* (MRSA) and *Clostridium difficile* (C. diff), that are largely hospital based. The Ebola scare offers a vivid illustration of the kind of thing hospitals must look out for. What has become clear, is that the antibiotics needed to overcome the infections must be developed at a faster rate because newer and more virulent super bugs keep appearing at a steadily increasing rate. Hospitals are expected to be more vigilant in controlling hospital-based infections and are now penalized for not doing so.

GROWTH AND DEVELOPMENT

By the middle of the twentieth century people were not only more willing to go into the hospital, they were prepared to stay there for days.

However, even at that time, staying in the hospital was not a minor expense. So who paid for people to luxuriate in the hospital for days? The answer is health insurance, initially Blue Cross, later commercial insurance, and as of 1966, Medicare and Medicaid. (See chapters 5 and 6 for more detailed discussion of health insurance.)

The enactment of Medicare and Medicaid turned out to be a huge event for the future of hospitals and health care in general in this country. The two programs guaranteed payment on behalf of persons who had been least likely to be hospitalized because they could not afford it. That brought in a lot of "new business" to hospitals, causing hospitals to grow and expand to accommodate increasing demand for health care services. (If talk about the business of health care delivery makes you think that things are finally going to be orderly and efficient, you're going to like what happens over the next few decades; if talk about the health care business makes you uncomfortable, prepare yourself, this is just the beginning. Hospitals and health care organizations are about to become BIG BUSINESS. Remember how much we are spending on hospital care?)

From the perspective of hospitals, Medicare, and to a lesser extent Medicaid, plus private insurance would be providing a steady stream of funding from this time forward. The government wanted some assurance that government funds would be going to good, as opposed to fly-by-night, hospitals. Therefore, the government decreed that Medicare funds could only go to hospitals accredited by the Joint Commission (remember this is the voluntary association created to upgrade standards). Hospitals that could not successfully pass a review by the Joint Commission closed because they could not compete with hospitals that were eager to emphasize that they had received this stamp of approval in the literature they produced to describe themselves.

HOSPITAL BILLING

Policy makers who participated in designing the Medicare and Medicaid legislation reasoned that a backlog of untreated illness would push up the initial costs of Medicare and Medicaid but that once that backlog was addressed costs would drop. It did not take long to find that expenditures were not dropping. They were continuing to go up. The government did not take major steps to reduce Medicare costs associated with hospital care, until 1983, when Diagnostic Related Groups (DRGs) were introduced. The government developed a reimbursement schedule based on the diagnoses with which patients were admitted to the hospital and the treatments that followed. Hospitals were fully aware that this was coming and knew that the government was using the data that the hospitals themselves were submitting in order to receive Medicare reimbursements. Amazingly, all possible diagnostic categories were subsumed into 467 categories, plus a few more catchall categories. The system was set up so that the government would pay X amount of money per diagnostic category (1 of the 467; that number has grown to about 750) per Medicare patient admission. While private insurance companies adopted the DRG categorizations, they reimbursed hospitals at a higher rate than Medicare.

The introduction of DRGs marked an important turning point in the operation of hospitals. Consider the fact that, prior to DRGs, Medicare and all other insurers paid hospitals based on *charges, not costs*. In other words, whatever the hospital charged was what insurers paid. Critics repeatedly pointed out that paying on a charge, rather than cost, basis was one of the main reasons behind the escalation of costs. They argued that hospitals could and should become more efficient and accountable for how they were spending public funds. The government took steps to encourage hospitals to become more efficient by announcing that it would standardize reimbursements. If the hospital could do whatever was necessary for less than the DRG payment for particular procedures or services, it got to keep the extra funds. If the funds were insufficient, the hospital simply had to find a way to do it. Hospitals came up with various ways to deal with it. One was to increase charges to patients covered by private insurance. Another way was to begin cutting back on the number of days (*length of stay*) a person stayed in the hospital. In 1980, people were staying in the hospital an average of 7.5 days; by 2010, they were staying 4.8 days.[4] It is also true that patients have less risk of acquiring a hospital-based infection and getting more rest if they stay for a shorter time.

Hospitals instituted another tactic that turned out to be very successful in making up for lost earnings. They were already reducing the length of stay—all they had to do was extend that idea. They simply admitted patients for less than a full day (i.e., less than twenty-four hours). Since DRGs cover *inpatient* care but not *outpatient* care, hospitals could charge rates that were not so closely monitored for treating patients on an outpatient basis. Hospitals began building freestanding outpatient clinics both near and far from the parent hospital.

To deal with health care delivered outside of the hospital, in clinics owned by hospitals, Medicare in conjunction with the AHA created a new reimbursement schedule. This is known as the Healthcare Common Procedure Coding System (HCPCS). If you are a stickler for detail, you are going to like the following "alphabet soup" explanation. The HCPSC code is built on the CPT (Current Procedural Terminology) code created by the AMA. Centers for Medicare and Medicaid Services (CMS) assigns a Level I HCPSC code for every medical, surgical, and diagnostic procedure carried out in a hospital; Level II codes cover all items and supplies not covered by Level I. The HCPSC code is also used by organizations and agencies (e.g., AMA, JCAHO) for data collection purposes. There is more. In order to make U.S. statistics comparable to international statistics, hospitals are required to report mortality and morbidity data using International Statistical Classification of Diseases (ICD) codes. The codes have been revised numerous times and are now in the ICD-10 phase. Hospitals must adopt the ICD-10 schedule by October 2015. They have resisted doing so because of the cost and turmoil that reorganizing billing procedures brings.

The U.S. Centers for Disease Control and Prevention (CDC) uses ICD codes (not CPT codes) in reporting international data. All the coding measures have their own manuals, which are updated regularly. In addition, a number of committees have been established to advise on updating each set of codes. It is no wonder that training courses are offered by any number of organizations to train people seeking to become coders.

At about the time DRGs were introduced, a number of other factors came into play that contributed to further reducing the length of stay in the hospital. Surgical techniques had been improving all along, more laser surgery was being used (which is less invasive and may be done on an outpatient basis), and, as we noted earlier, everyone agrees that it is better for the patient to go home to more familiar and comforting surroundings. Length of stay has a big impact on hospital *occupancy rates*. If people stay in the hospital for fewer days, that leaves beds empty. If this trend continues hospitals have to take beds out of service

permanently. That is exactly what happened. The effect of the introduction of DRGs is that some hospitals had such a low "census" or occupancy rate that they could no longer survive.

The upshot of this trend is that hospitals were now admitting more
patients who were too seriously ill to be treated on an outpatient basis.
This manifested itself in two diametrically opposed trends that actually
make perfect sense when you think about it. First, hospitals had no
alternative but to increase the ratio of staff to patients; second, personnel costs were steadily declining compared to other hospital costs,
which were skyrocketing. What accounts for rising hospital costs is not
so difficult to understand once you realize how much new technology
hospitals were investing in. This includes diagnostic and monitoring
equipment like CT (computerized axial tomography) scanners, MRI
(magnetic resonance imaging) equipment, PET (positron emission tomography) scanners, and the computers that compile and analyze all
the information that the diagnostic equipment produces. All those machines are enormously expensive, and they are replaced every few years
as newer, improved versions are released. Of course, every patient
wants the most recent version of any diagnostic instrument available,
and your doctor certainly feels that way, too; that, among other things
(like the threat of malpractice suits for using outdated equipment),
convinces the hospital that staying current is a wise investment.

In order to cover these costs, hospitals increasingly began relying on
a very old and familiar funding mechanism, namely, the "sliding scale,"
meaning the rich pay more. In its more recent incarnation, it became
known as "cost-shifting," that is, charging privately insured patients
more than those whose bills were paid by public insurance, because
public insurance programs reimburse hospitals at a lower rate than
private insurance and make every effort to monitor those expenditures.

Unfair? Hospital representatives say that they must take care of persons who carry no insurance but run up high costs. Where are they
supposed to get the funds to cover that? Laws passed in 1986 prevent
hospitals from turning away patients who are uninsured and unable to
pay for care. Therefore, people who had no other regular source of care
began coming to emergency rooms with minor as well as major problems, because they knew they would not be turned away even if they
could not pay for the care they received.

Hospitals are allowed to stabilize the patients who cannot pay for their care in the emergency room before sending them off, ideally to the nearest "safety net" hospital. However, this sometimes involves emergency surgery and days spent in the most expensive part of the hospital, the "intensive care" unit. Surgical patients who are admitted to the hospital for a planned, routine surgery typically only spend a short period of time there. Patients who are involved in serious accidents or have multiple gunshot wounds stay much longer.

The recession has had a rather dramatic effect on hospitals. According to the Agency for Healthcare Research and Quality (AHRQ), which operates under the auspices of the HHS, hospital stays for uninsured patients increased by 21 percent between 2003 and 2008.[5] By contrast, the total increase in hospital stays was 4 percent. Can you see why the hospital sector would be interested in seeing health care reform passed that would reduce the chances that uninsured people would require hospitalization?

This brings us back to "bad debt," the amount of money the hospital loses when it cares for uninsured persons or provides services that third party payers do not cover. (Remember nonprofit hospitals have to have a plan outlining the care they will provide for a nonprofit designation excusing them from federal taxes. Bad debt does not accomplish that.) What constitutes bad debt is worth looking at more closely. A few years ago, Congress asked the Government Accounting Organization (GAO) to examine how hospitals calculate "bad debt." The GAO concluded that a single measure does not exist.

As an aside: The government reimburses hospitals at the rate of 65 percent for bad debt. Where the bad debt number comes from is absolutely astounding. Get ready for a pretty amazing story about how this works. Every hospital has something called a "chargemaster." This is the price list for all goods and services the hospital provides, down to a single aspirin. It can run to 10,000 items. The hospital issues a bill based on its chargemaster price list. Hospitals treat the part of the hospital bill—based on the chargemaster price list—that is not covered by the patient or patient's insurance as bad debt. The really interesting thing is that each hospital comes up with its own prices for all of the items on the list. The prices do not look like the prices any other hospital charges for the same things. And there is no requirement for hospitals to make this public—to anyone. The only state that requires hospitals to make the chargemaster list public is California. Analysts have been having a great time studying the lists submitted by California hospitals, comparing them from one hospital to another and speculating about the lists in other states. We will get back to this point, when we get to health care system reform later in this chapter.

Hospitals have been creative in dealing with the imposition of increased efforts on the part of the government to control costs. Hospitals have been buying and consolidating physician practice groups. This allows hospitals to bill for medical services delivered by affiliated doctors. This has given hospitals a great degree of leverage in dealing with insurance companies and purchasing agreements with organizations that provide all kinds of products used by hospitals.

GROWTH OF THE FOR-PROFIT HOSPITAL SECTOR

Policy experts became interested in the effects of the steady expansion of for-profit hospitals several decades ago. The representatives of the for-profit hospital corporations argued that what they were doing was socially beneficial because it put pressure on nonprofit hospitals to be more efficient, which, they said, would bring down prices. Critics countered by arguing that the for-profit hospital corporations employed tactics that deserved greater scrutiny. And that closer scrutiny indicates that the for-profit hospitals are not necessarily more efficient. As we noted earlier, the new suburban for-profit hospitals that have been increasing in number generally care for patients who are less seriously ill. They simply charge more, provide less charitable care, operate with lower patient-staff ratios, and do little or no research. They have lower personnel costs, which they achieve by replacing nurses with advanced training by hiring less expensive, easily replaced "technicians" to do very specific tasks. The technicians take blood pressure or give "shots." The idea was to employ a factory model breaking down tasks so that a person could be easily trained to carry a particular task. When some of the nonprofit hospitals tried this tactic they found that bringing in less skilled personnel increases the risk of mistakes—medication errors, inability to recognize indicators that something is not right, carelessness about disposal of infectious materials, and so on. Why the new for-profit hospitals could take advantage of this tactic is that the hospitals were being built in areas where they would attract patients more likely to require routine, less complicated, and less costly, care. This is in contrast to the problems that urban hospitals are more likely to see coming through the doors of their emergency rooms. In fact, suburban for-profit hospitals are less likely to have emergency rooms.

The larger problem, according to some observers, was that the new more aggressive business practices introduced by the for-profit hospital chains eventually led to mergers and buyouts of smaller hospitals. The hospital corporations were acting like other businesses. Critics maintained that the for-profits were skimming off the richest, healthiest patients, were doing almost no research, no medical education, and had as their primary goal financial gain benefiting hospital executives and shareholders. They went on to argue that the health care delivery system should not be making a profit on the members of society who have the misfortune of being sick. When the FBI charged two of the leading for-profit chains with fraud and very publicly raided their offices during the early years of the twenty-first century—for overcharging Medicare and performing unnecessary surgery—critics said that no one should be surprised because the for-profit approach manifested such behavior. (For a graphic account, see Marcia Mahar's *Money-Driven Medicine*.[6])

Nonprofit hospitals did take notice of the advice they were being given by some policy makers who were pressing the nonprofits to act more like for-profits—to use business practices and become more efficient. Larger, more well-established nonprofit hospitals began to buy up smaller hospitals. They formed networks. They incorporated, but remained nonprofit organizations. They gained a major bargaining advantage in dealing with suppliers, including insurance companies. They were now in a position to negotiate with insurance companies, offering lower charges in exchange for having the insurance company funnel all its enrollees to that hospital network. Insurance companies have been known to complain that the networked hospitals, both for-profit and nonprofit, have attained an unfair negotiating advantage.

Patients who get care outside of the network linked to their health insurance plan are charged the full fee. As you can imagine, patients who find themselves in this situation are generally outraged by the size of the bill. Hospitals are typically willing to negotiate the bill, but the patient must request the reduction in charges. There are no rules governing how this is worked out.

OTHER HEALTH CARE ORGANIZATIONS

Applying one of the basic differentiating characteristics that we used in discussing hospitals, we can differentiate some other health care organizations by whether they care for patients who are *ambulatory* (to ambulate is to walk) or *bedridden*. Ambulatory patients may receive care at clinics, now more often called health centers, which can be freestanding or attached to a hospital. They can be acutely (but temporarily) ill or chronically ill; in both cases they receive health care services on an outpatient basis, for whatever time it takes, meaning a long-term or short-term basis. Persons who may not really be sick but are no longer able to get to the hospital or clinic on a regular basis without a great deal of assistance may end up being admitted to a facility to receive care as inpatients.

Health centers located in poor communities receive support from the Health Resources and Services Administration (HRSA), an agency created during the Carter administration, operating under the auspices of HHS. HRSA provides funding through grants for which the health center must apply to become designated a Federally Qualified Health Center (FQHC). The centers must show that they are serving a medically underserved population in a particular community that may include migrant workers, homeless residents, or residents of public housing. Centers that meet the criteria for this designation but have not applied for it are known as look-alike centers. They qualify for some of the benefits but not all.

Such centers must be governed by a community board representing the population being served. The centers must have a sliding scale fee system in place based on family size and income. The FQHC designation comes with certain benefits. For example, they may purchase drugs at reduced cost, vaccines are provided for uninsured children at no cost, and the centers serve as sites where National Health Service Corps (NHSC) medical, dental, and mental health providers may work and receive educational loan repayment (up to $170,000) at no cost to the centers, and providers who work there are provided malpractice insurance by the federal government. FQHCs seem to be doing exactly what they were created to do. Is everyone satisfied to see this happening? Not exactly. Most analysts agree that the FQHCs work well. It is just that there is no assurance that they are being formed in all the places where they are needed. Distribution is unsystematic because it is voluntary and depends on community initiative and capability, which vary a lot for any number of reasons, density, for example.

Turning to long-term care facilities, we find that long-term care has been attracting a considerable amount of attention for some time as the baby boom generation came ever closer to its golden years. As we have already noted, that time has finally arrived with 2011 marking the first year that baby boomers turned sixty-five. And as we have also noted, as the boomers develop health problems associated with aging they are expected to break the bank; and that the list of threatened institutions is lengthy: social security, Medicare, nursing homes, and all associated services required by the elderly.

Added to the increasing number of people who will need nursing home care because of the problems associated with aging, there is the devastation that chronic illness in younger populations causes, for example, developmental disabilities, paralysis due to spinal injury, mental problems, and so forth. Finally, the fact that modern medicine can perform miracles in saving people who would not have survived years ago does not necessarily mean that those who are saved can lead normal, healthy lives. Many require extensive care for years.

Home health care has been supported, in fact promoted, albeit with some trepidation, by the government as a good alternative to nursing home care. The reason that home health care is not likely to be promoted even more enthusiastically is that it poses a potential cost problem that is interesting to reflect upon. Home health care is much less expensive than nursing home care because people stay in their own homes and health workers go in for a few hours at a time. Also, virtually everyone prefers to stay in his or her own home. The fear is that too many people will opt for this form of care. Traditionally, wives, daughters, and other female relatives provided such care out of a sense of duty. Now that the majority of women are not staying home, the government is concerned that it will have to pick up the bill. For now, the costs do not seem to be rising too rapidly but this cost item is being carefully monitored.

Hospices are another interesting innovation. For years, critics said terminally ill patients did not have to be in the hospital. It was too expensive; it put the patient through unnecessary pain and aggravation; it was a bad idea all around. Hospices promised to provide the patient with comfort and relief from pain, rather than aggressive intervention. The result was expected to be less expensive. As it turns out, the kind of care patients are receiving is pretty much what was anticipated. Most people think it is excellent. The problem is that it has not reduced costs very much.

One of the problems that comes up repeatedly is that HHS inspectors keep finding nursing homes in violation of federal health and safety standards. The homes owned by for-profit chains are consistently found to have more violations than either the nonprofit or government-owned nursing homes.[7] The fact that about two-thirds are owned by for-profit companies, 27 percent are nonprofit, and 6 percent are government owned is, according to some observers, the reason behind the high rate of violations being reported.

HOSPITALS AND HEALTH CARE REFORM

Hospitals have been expanding in preparation for the influx of newly insured patients in response to ACA mandates. While the ACA promised increased hospital income, it was also expected to bring clearly specified payment reductions tied to quality of care.

Medicare has developed a list of "never events" announcing that hospitals will not be reimbursed for inpatient stays when such events occur. Examples of never events include surgery on the wrong site, wrong procedure given the diagnosis, leaving something inside the patient during surgery, allowing a serious infection to develop at the site of the surgery, and an excessive rate of readmissions within 30 days post-hospitalization, to name a few such events. Policy analysts have expressed concern that there has been a serious undercounting of adverse events even after enactment of the ACA.[8] A study, authored by surgeons focusing on surgical errors, reported that there are nearly eighty surgical errors per week; in some cases they found temporary harm, but in one-third of the cases they found permanent harm.[9]

Preventable error is a serious matter. It has obvious implications for patient health and safety. It also has cost implications. According to one assessment, the top ten preventable errors account for over two-thirds of the $17.1 billion in costs associated with such errors.[10] Reports on mechanisms designed to identify and track hospital error continue to attract attention. [11] The AHRQ has recently issued a statement outlining the steps hospitals can take to improve quality. [12] It is interesting to see that the statement is titled "10 Patient Safety Tips for Hospitals." (My point is that government agencies are careful about issuing statements saying that health care providers "should" do something unless there are regulations in place. The AHRQ's statement is clearly identified as advice.)

Another mechanism CMS has instituted is making public a lot of the information it collects. Based on information gathered by the Hospital Quality Alliance (HQA), CMS created a consumer-oriented web site called Hospital Compare that reports hospital errors. It released its first report in March 2011. The HQA is a public-private collaboration that involves a wide range of organizations, including organizations that represent consumers, hospitals, employers, accrediting groups, and doctors in addition to federal agencies. The value of the report depends on the accuracy of the information. Hospitals have identified errors in the reports but generally agree that assessment serves as a useful tool that helps to pinpoint problems. Whether patients are accessing this information is another question.

The fact that the ACA has issued a directive requiring hospitals to submit their chargemaster pricing lists to their respective state agencies means that reimbursement rates will receive scrutiny from various interested parties, including payers. This is expected to have a sizable effect on costs. It is not exactly clear when this will occur.

One other feature of the ACA can be expected to have a significant and lasting impact. Hospitals have been encouraged to form Accountable Care Organizations (ACOs) in cooperation with networks of doctors. The ACO must enroll a minimum of five thousand Medicare patients before it can go on to enroll other patients. The incentive for creating an ACO is the bonus payment it receives from Medicare for holding down costs, meeting certain benchmarks for care, and keeping patients out of the hospital. By the end of 2014, there were more than 600 ACOs. There are more ACOs in some states than others.

Another restriction included in the ACA is the prohibition against creation of new specialty hospitals. The intent, at least in part, is cost reduction. Specialty hospitals were being established by doctors for the purpose of treating a specific health problem. The trend started in 2000 when doctors began promoting a "focused factory" approach to treatment. The quality of care they were delivering was, with few exceptions, found to be excellent; patients were highly satisfied. So what's the problem? Community hospital administrators claimed that physicians were referring insured, less complicated cases to facilities in which they had a financial interest. This was placing a greater burden on community hospitals to care for the more complicated cases and uninsured patients. At last count there were two hundred specialty hospitals in existence.

It is fair to conclude that hospitals were not the primary target of health care reform. However, the introduction of a "bundling" payment system is expected to have a major impact. Hospitals may choose from four bundled payment options offered by Medicare covering inpatient, outpatient, continued care, or some mix of these. The objective is moving away from fee-for-service reimbursement. Hospitals that manage to deliver care at a cost lower than the bundled payment keep those funds and receive a bonus for their efficiency. Major teaching hospitals have been more willing to sign on than other hospitals.

The mandates handed down by the ACA that affect hospitals certainly address two of the three health systems goals, namely quality and cost control. Aiming to increase access to hospital care requires other measures, mainly providing patients with the ability to pay for hospital care. How much of an impact the ACA has on the steps hospitals take to improve quality, contain costs, and increase access is something that should keep policy analysts busy for years to come.

QUESTIONS AND ISSUES TO THINK ABOUT

- Given what you now know about the hospital sector, what indicators would you use to determine whether hospitals are achieving a measure of success in controlling costs and improving the quality of care?
- Let's consider efficiency. Government hospitals are regularly said to be inefficient. Although most people can't tell the difference between nonprofit and for-profit hospitals, now that you know the difference, would you conclude that for-profit hospitals are more efficient than government hospitals? More efficient than nonprofit hospitals? What are the criteria you are using to make these assessments?

- Hospitals buy a lot of very expensive high-tech equipment such as CT scanners and MRIs. This adds a lot to national health costs. Would imposing controls over which hospitals can buy such equipment be worth considering? Or would that be detrimental? If so, in what way would it be detrimental?

4

HEALTH CARE OCCUPATIONS

This chapter focuses on health care occupations, how they developed, and how they have changed over time. The closing section of the chapter outlines how passage of the health care reform act affects health occupations.

The number of people involved in the delivery of health care and the tasks they perform have been steadily increasing. The Bureau of Labor Statistics (BLS) reports that as of 2011, nearly 11 percent of all the jobs in this country are in the health sector. Consider this figure in contrast to what the health sector looked like a century ago. It is not much of an exaggeration to say that at the beginning of the twentieth century, there were only three positions in the hospital: doctor, nurse, and aide. The doctors' job was to diagnose and treat the patient. Nurses were responsible for keeping the patient clean and comfortable; aides, who may not have been called aides at the time, dealt with household work. Doctors' offices had no support staff. Sometimes, the doctor's wife would help with the bills, and someone had to clean the office. How things have changed! Furthermore, this is one of the few parts of the labor force that is predicted to continue expanding, that is, employing even more people in the foreseeable future. Which raises a number of basic questions, such as: Where did all those jobs come from? Who is in charge of creating new jobs? How does the work get divided up?

Some 450 occupational titles are involved. Obviously we can only discuss a small number of them. We will devote most attention to doctors, because doctors have the final authority when it comes to diagnosis and treatment. This is an exclusive right of doctors, with a few notable exceptions such as advanced practice nurses, including nurse practitioners, nurse anesthetists, and nurse midwives. Practice privileges vary from state to state. A number of other occupational groups have been challenging doctors' exclusive right to prescribe and treat patients. We will return to this topic in chapter 9.

THE MEDICAL PROFESSION

Let's go back to the late nineteenth century to see how medicine as an occupation developed. A number of explanations competed for the existence of ill health, even death, all represented by groups of practitioners who offered a particular set of treatments based on those explanations. There were many kinds of practitioners: hydropaths (who used water to soothe, but more often than not to aggressively heat up or cool down the body); naturopaths (who use natural herbal preparations in prevention and treatment of symptoms); chiropractors (who treat most ailments using back manipulation and massage); homeopaths (who believe in treating "like symptoms with like" in an effort to attain stability and bring comfort); osteopaths or DOs (doctors of osteopathy, who subscribe to the idea that the backbone is the body's control center and that its strength is central to good health); and, allopaths (who engaged in aggressive interventions, such as bloodletting and giving emeties to induce vomiting, and if they were not successful, they simply applied more of the same treatment, but were the ones who ultimately succeeded in laying the foundation for mainstream medicine).

By the beginning of the twentieth century, allopathic medicine had firmly allied itself with medical science. The other practitioners did not exactly disappear, although some were absorbed by allopathic, mainstream medicine while others came to be defined as unscientific and lost ground. Practitioners other than mainstream medical doctors now offer what has been called "alternative medicine" or, more recently, "complementary" and "integrative" medicine. The scientific community does not deny that complementary medicine may provide benefits. It is just that the diagnoses and treatments are so individualized that they cannot be standardized or confirmed. What works for one person may not work the same way for another person. Moreover, the medications are not regulated by the Food and Drug Administration. The result is that, as one investigation after another reveals with considerable fanfare, the amount of active ingredient in the medications may or may not be accurate, and may not even be there at all. Yet some people continue to swear by these products and until a scandal occurs, severe injury or death of a number of people, no one demands that better controls be instituted. And after a while, the whole issue dies down again.

What is it about allopathic medicine that is different, that made it scientific? And why did that allow the allopaths to win the battle of competing explanations for illness and death (i.e., morbidity and mortality, respectively)? Being "scientific" simply means that the explanations and, ultimately, the treatments allopathic medicine was offering at the end of the nineteenth century could be substantiated. The allopaths could predict the course of disease with and without treatment. The same was true from one instance or one person to another. They verified their diagnoses by doing autopsies. This allowed doctors to compare the symptoms outlined in the patient's file to the effect on the organs involved. They built up a body of knowledge and learned to apply it. An increasing number of people began to believe in their explanations as evidence of their success began to accumulate. Or, if you prefer, the allopaths made every effort to make sure people heard about their successes and were impressed by them.

The larger context of the times in which all this was taking place is worth reflecting on for a moment. This was happening at about the same time that Americans had suddenly become convinced that science was the way to go in all areas of life. During the first decade of the twentieth century there was talk about scientific solutions for such unlikely pursuits as housewifery (i.e., housekeeping) and such popular ones (in some circles) as scientific management. The growth of confidence in scientific medicine was not a unique phenomenon but rather a part of a broader shift in social values and expectations.

Accordingly, when the allopaths (hereafter referred to as doctors or MDs) focused on one area of practice, that is, chose to specialize in treatment of that part of the body, they received high praise and recognition. Patients who could afford it were eager to be treated by medical specialists. True, the vast majority of people could not afford the kind of care medical experts could provide. They relied on home remedies and elixirs provided by the corner druggist. Preference for treatment by specialists was something the social elite could indulge in and the middle class made every effort to emulate, and which the poor pretty much ignored because they could not afford to be treated by a doctor, let alone a specialist.

MEDICAL SPECIALIZATION

Let's consider the matter of specialization in more detail. It is worth going back to the late nineteenth and early twentieth centuries again in order to get the full picture. The first specialty to emerge was ophthalmology (medical and surgical treatment of the eye). One reason for this might be that new and better tools were becoming available during the latter half of the nineteenth century, making it easier to detect abnormalities in the eye. By the late 1800s small groups of doctors were meeting to discuss their observations about the eye and the new tools they were just getting accustomed to using. They were the ones who decided to establish a specialty of their own. Why do that? Was the chance to make more money a primary motivation here? A closer look at how people entered into most occupations might help answer that question.

At the turn of the century one announced his or her occupation by putting up a sign declaring the kinds of work he (mostly he) was prepared to do. City directories, which were much like (our fast disappearing) telephone books, listed people's occupations. You could list any occupation you wanted, qualified or not. People could, and did, simply pick up, move, and start doing different kinds of work whenever it suited them. This might be surprising but, until the last decades of the nineteenth century, there was strong opposition to all forms of licensure. When the movement to institute licensure took hold in the 1880s, it occurred on a state-by-state basis. Today states continue to control licensure, and a license from one state may not be honored in another state.

Returning to our ophthalmology example, why would an individual be interested in developing an official specialty designation? After all, anyone who had a medical degree, and, in some cases, those who did not, could put up a sign saying that they specialized in treating diseases of the eye. Conversely, no one would want to let just anybody treat their

eyes. But wasn't insisting that practitioners be required to have a medical license enough? People wanted to be assured that they were going
to practitioners who really had the best skills at the time when it came
to treating something like the eye. The doctors who were restricting
their practices to treating people's eye problems and meeting with colleagues to upgrade their knowledge on a regular basis did in fact know
more about eye disease than anyone else. They actually did have greater
expertise in their field, but there was no sure way for them to distinguish themselves from anyone else who laid claim to the label of eye
specialist.

It was the experts in treatment of eye diseases who decided to institute specialty "certification." The doctors themselves set up training
programs and a qualifying test for the purpose of recognizing new practitioners as qualified specialists. Thus, in 1916, ophthalmology became
the first certified specialty. Other areas of specialization followed. However, the majority of doctors continued to identify themselves as general
practitioners throughout the first half of the twentieth century.

As an aside, how do you think other physicians reacted to the emergence of certification in ophthalmology? They were generally pleased,
as most reputable doctors were not interested in treating eye problems
because the eye is such a complex organ.

World War II stands as a major turning point in how medicine developed in this country, including specialized medicine. The wartime
draft made a major impression on doctors. Specialists entered into military service as captains while the general practitioners entered as lieu-
tenants. Obviously, with the higher rank of captain came higher pay and
other privileges. Not the least of the privileges was the fact that captains
were assigned to hospitals away from the battleground, while the lieu-
tenants were assigned to field hospitals at the front.

A related trend was taking off at home. Because wartime wages were
frozen, the only way that companies could make themselves more attractive to prospective employees, who were in short supply, was to
offer better benefits. Insurance companies could not operate without
making some effort to standardize the fees they would pay for the
medical services. Prior to this time, doctors pretty much decided what
to charge depending on where they practiced and how much their
patients were able to pay. Insurance companies agreed to permit specialists to charge higher fees than general practitioners.

Once the war ended, there is the effect of the GI Bill to consider. One of the big rewards for military service during the war was free education upon return. A large number of veterans took advantage of this benefit, including those who already had an MD degree. They went on to get more education and experience better suited to treating patients who were not war casualties. With more training, they became eligible for certification as specialists. Some went on to take specialty certification exams. Many others announced that they were specialists based on the fact that they completed all the requirements and were qualified to take certification tests even if they did not actually take that final step. How did society react? People were eager to be treated by doctors who had the most knowledge and expertise, that is, those who were trained as specialists.

Continuing to take a historical perspective, we find that the central feature of life in the United States from the mid-1960s through the early 1970s, in addition to the Vietnam War, antiwar protests, and the civil rights movement, was the increased role that the government was playing in civilian life. The government was funneling considerable sums of money into programs of all kinds—education, housing, social welfare—with medical research receiving a fair share of those funds. Research monies went to medical schools for the purpose of performing specific kinds of research. There was an explosion of scientific knowledge. Medical students were not at all sure that they could learn everything they needed to know. Specialization allowed them to learn more about one subject area. Furthermore, medical students were heavily influenced by the excitement surrounding the work of specialists and super-specialists. Medical faculty served as impressive role models for new trainees. [1]

As an aside, this is important in understanding why we continue to see some doctors being more aggressive in ordering tests and prescribing treatment while other doctors take a more "wait and see" approach. We come back to the variation in practice patterns in chapter 8 to discuss the impact this has on the cost of care.

In the meantime, with all the emphasis on specialization, general practitioners were becoming unhappy. They were being paid less than specialists for providing many of the same services. Patients were referring themselves to specialists because they perceived specialists to be more knowledgeable. The general practitioners decided that they were tired of being treated like second-class citizens. They decided to make themselves specialists in "family practice." In 1971, family practice became a specialty just like any other medical or surgical specialty. After finishing medical school and receiving their MDs, doctors continued their training in specialized residency programs. Prior to this time, a person with an MD was required to complete a one-year internship program in order to obtain a license to practice, granted by the state. From 1971 on, all MDs would be required to complete residencies lasting at least three years, more to become even more highly specialized. In short, as of 1971, MDs could no longer become general practitioners. Doctors receiving the Doctor of Osteopathy degree, DOs, have increasingly been serving as the country's general practitioners. Some DOs have gone on for specialty training by entering residency programs offered by MD medical schools.

We now refer to doctors who are primarily responsible for monitoring a patient's health as "primary care" practitioners. This includes internists, pediatricians, and family practitioners.

MEDICAL ERROR AND MALPRACTICE

Coincidentally, just about the time that the general practice option was abolished, Americans began to register increasing dissatisfaction with their health care arrangements. They complained that doctors were no longer interested in the whole person; that they were only interested in treating parts of the person; and that they were only doing it for the money. Why this did not happen previously when doctors could do so much less for their patients is not hard to understand when you consider that over previous decades, the majority of doctors were general practitioners who were located in the community where their patients lived. Members of the community got to know the doctor. When they needed to see the doctor, they went with the added comfort of an established sense of familiarity and trust. That is not the case when patients see a specialist for a specific problem on a one-time basis. When things go wrong, it is a lot easier to sue that doctor, who is, after all, a stranger. This explains, in part, the high rate at which patients have been suing doctors for malpractice.

A number of other factors, including the rising size of settlements, may have contributed to what has come to be viewed as a malpractice crisis during the early years of the twenty-first century. Some observers believe that the widely quoted report on the rate of medical error has something to do with it. The matter of medical error came to public attention in 1999 when the Institute of Medicine reported that 44,000 to 98,000 people die in hospitals per year due to preventable error.[2] While the numbers were actively disputed, everyone agreed that error reduction was a highly laudable objective. Interest in the issue contin- ues in conjunction with efforts to improve quality of care. New tools designed to identify error find a higher rate of error.

The IOM report clearly stated that the rate of error was due to systemic failure rather than malpractice on the part of doctors. The fact that the public media chose to focus on the failure of doctors rather than systemic failure in covering the report may have prompted some patients to sue.

There is no reliable count of the number of malpractice suits that are filed per year, their outcome, or the awards. Researchers who have studied this issue focus largely on the impact malpractice has had on health care spending.[3] The costs include the time and expense of deal- ing with the suits, legal expenses, the awards. Beyond that, doctors argue that they are forced to practice defensive medicine. That means that they order tests they know are not really necessary in order to avoid the accusation that they did not do everything possible to treat the patient.

At least fifteen states have no limits on the amount of money that can be awarded in a malpractice suit. Others have imposed varying limits. However, it is the award for "pain and suffering" that is most controversial. Awards for costs of treatment and lost wages are generally not disputed. There is no definition of pain and suffering, so juries receive no instruction regarding appropriate awards, which results in enormous variation. The pain and suffering award is an addition to actual expenditures and costs. A blog authored by Michael Krauss in *Forbes*, a business-oriented publication, on April 17, 2014, illustrates the point.

> A 40-year-old woman gave birth to a healthy and loved (by her own admission) baby after a failed tubal ligation [a contraception proce-

dure], and sued her OB-GYN for damages. . . . The jury found the doctor liable and found economic damages of $39,000 for medical expenses (the cost of birthing) and $9,000 in Mom's lost wages . . . $48,000. . . . Yet the total award was $1,800,000, meaning that $1,752,000 was awarded for pain and suffering—for a baby that was loved and perfectly healthy (and a happy 6-year-old at the time of the jury verdict).

In another case

A woman with multiple allergies . . . provided a list of her known drug allergies . . . and was administered an inhaled steroid to which she had a known allergy. . . . Ten days' [sic] hospitalization ensued. When the patient left the hospital she could not swallow solid foods and could not recline. Her voice was hoarse, her hair fell out, and she had two surgeries to correct laryngeal scarring and tracheal narrowing. She was out of work for six months. She had economic damages of $43,000 in lost wages and $97,000 in medical and hospital fees, for a total of $140,000. She agreed to a settlement of $627,868 including therefore roughly $387,000 for pain and suffering. Clearly the plaintiff's competent counsel feared recovering less before the jury; otherwise she would not have settled for this amount.

The author sums up these examples by saying: "It's hard to avoid the 'tort lottery' conclusion here. 'Tort lottery' and 'equal justice before the law' don't go together well." He goes on to discuss the variation in malpractice premiums. In California, which is the first state to institute a cap of $250,000 on pain and suffering awards, OB-GYNs pay $50,000 for malpractice insurance. Recent estimates indicate that they pay $140,000 in Chicago and $175,000 in Long Island. Illinois and New York do not have a cap on pain and suffering awards.

It should not be surprising to hear that lawyers are opposed to tort reform. They argue that suing doctors is the best approach for protecting patients from incompetent doctors because the threat of being penalized makes doctors more careful. Doctors argue that lawyers are motivated to sue even when there is no evidence of error because they stand to collect one-third of the settlement if they go to court and win and one-fourth if the case is settled out of court. They take cases on "contingency," that is, they get paid only if they win and get paid nothing if they lose. Lawyers say that this allows people who could not possibly afford to hire a lawyer and pay all the costs involved in a trial to be represented.

For their part, insurance companies are willing to settle out of court on a batch of suits without expending the resources required to determine whether there is evidence of medical error and the extent of the error. Insurance companies do this to avoid the cost of going to court. The settlements, in turn, raise malpractice premium costs for all doctors in the insurance pool and leave an undeserved blemish on doctors' records whose cases were settled without any effort to check to see whether the claims had any validity to them. Some doctors have countersued and won. However, that takes more time, money, and aggravation than most are willing to invest.

What do policy makers say is the most promising solution for reducing the risk of malpractice? Many argue that the solution is continued medical education for doctors and safety checklists for hospitals. Safety checklists have had a major effect on reduction of hospital-based error and infection. Counting instruments in the surgical suite before closing up the patient eliminates one clearly avoidable error. Hand washing and using hand sanitizers has had an enormous impact on reducing hospital-based infections, which are especially difficult to treat once patients are exposed to them. It is not difficult to see why policy analysts would argue that taking such steps produces significant social benefit and is probably a better way to deal with malpractice than other approaches. It is also a lot less controversial. (You might want to keep some of these points in mind; we will return to this subject in chapter 9.)

One more initiative, designed to reduce risk of mistakes related to paperwork if not medical practice, is based on shifting from paper to electronic medical record keeping. The Obama administration set aside $19 billion in the economic recovery act of 2009 to provide incentives for doctors to install electronic medical records software. The incentive came in the form of a $40,000 payment to physicians who initiate electronic record keeping. While most people agree this will help prevent prescription and treatment errors, it has been an uphill battle. The problems start with finding the right software, then getting everyone in the office trained to use it, then coordinating it with all the other offices, including hospital departments, and, finally, linking all this to billing. Because the choice of software has not been settled, getting the records linked is proving very troublesome. Eventually tracking patient treatment outcomes as well as billing will be made much more efficient, but this is not happening with lightning speed.

THE MEDICAL EDUCATION SYSTEM

Let's consider the historical development of medical schools in this country. As we have already discussed, prior to the twentieth century, anyone who was interested in setting up a medical practice could do so without the need to prove competence. This permitted a wide range of medical training arrangements, including apprenticeships with no coursework, no books, and no labs. Clearly, this was not the best way to learn about the practice of medicine. The "medical establishment" (that is code for organized medicine or the American Medical Association and its affiliates, the state and local medical societies) had been concerned about this situation ever since the middle of the nineteenth century when the AMA was established. However, the people who ran these inferior schools were colleagues and fellow AMA members. The issue was a delicate one. Most doctors weren't making a great deal of money treating patients, especially in communities that were not wealthy (remember there were no insurance companies that would guarantee payment in those days). Training fees were an important source of income. Telling colleagues that they would no longer be allowed to accept such fees because the schools they were operating were inferior was not a topic that other doctors wanted to broach.[4]

The situation was resolved without much input from the majority of people in society. The elite members of the AMA shared their concerns with others in their social circle, confident that such information would not be passed on to the wrong people (i.e., the public). This is when the Carnegie Foundation became interested in the problem. The Carnegie Foundation was (and still is) devoted to improving education at all levels. In 1907, it took on the task of improving the quality of medical education. The person who was invited to assume responsibility for this assignment was Abraham Flexner.

Flexner visited all 186 medical schools and training programs in existence at the time with the aim of rating them. He was welcomed because the Carnegie Foundation was known to distribute funds to schools. It was not until 1910, just before the Flexner Report was due to be released, that it became clear what Flexner was doing. He graded all the schools he visited on a scale of A through F. The schools to which he had given an "F" closed down even before the report was out. Others began upgrading immediately. Many could not survive. By 1920, only eighty medical schools were left.

The standard against which Flexner rated all other schools was the Johns Hopkins Medical School. He used Johns Hopkins as a model because it grounded its coursework in a scientific body of knowledge rather than in practical experience gained through apprenticeship. That meant two years of basic science courses before the school allowed students to see a patient under the supervision of a senior doctor. That is obviously an expensive proposition compared to apprenticeship training. It is easy to see why Johns Hopkins was not the first choice for those with limited resources.

The Flexner Report had a number of effects. It eliminated the worst medical schools, which were also the schools that prospective medical students from poor families could afford. That had an effect on the composition of the occupation. It had an effect on the chances of minority students being able to get a medical education. It affected women's medical schools, which lacked resources needed to upgrade. Few women were seeking a medical education in those days, and those who did generally did not come from wealthy families. Medicine also became more science-based. The smaller number of schools meant that fewer students could be accepted, which, in turn, meant that the schools could be more selective. The schools could accept only the most highly qualified applicants, who were, of course, white, male, and from a higher social class.

The quality of medical education is no longer a matter of major concern. The problem that policy makers have been most concerned about over recent decades is the cost of medical education and debt. According to the American Association of Medical Colleges (AAMC), physicians had an average educational debt in 2013–14 of $175,000. Another issue that has been receiving some attention is the need for more doctors. The AAMC is the leading voice calling for more doctors. (For more on this, see chapter 9.)

DOCTORS AND THE ISSUE OF MONEY

Given all the complaints about doctors, why is it that we as a society continue to pay them so much money? Let's look at how much they earn. In order to get a more detailed picture, let's look at the earnings of doctors in a sample of specialties. The figures are considerably larger for some subspecialties at the top of the income scale. Table 4.1 clearly illustrates the fact that there is a great deal of variation in the income by specialty.

Keep in mind that doctors' net income is considerably lower than their practice revenue because they must pay malpractice premiums and pay off educational loans. Would you agree that there is so much variation in earnings, it makes it harder to talk about doctors' income as if they all earn roughly the same amount? The ACA has instituted some adjustments intended to raise the compensation going to the three specialties at the bottom of the income scale.

There's more to the matter of how much doctors are reimbursed for their services. Something comparable to the DRG reimbursement arrangement for paying hospitals was created by the CMS in 1992 to standardize physician reimbursement, called the Resource Based Relative Value Scale (RBRVS). A team of economists from Harvard University worked it out in consultation with doctors and a variety of interested parties over a period of about four years. There were no surprises when it went into effect. The RBRVS schedule calculated a fee for every procedure that doctors perform as defined by the Current Procedural Terminology Code (CPT) created by the AMA. The AMA gives its

Table 4.1.   Physician Compensation

Discipline	Compensation (US$)
Orthopedics	421,000
Cardiology	376,000
Radiology	351,000
Internal Medicine	196,000
Family Medicine	195,000
Pediatrics	189,000

Source: Medscape Compensation Survey, 2015, http://www.medscape.com/features/slideshow/compensation/2015/public/overview#page=3.

recommendation for reimbursement to the Medicare Payment Adviso-ry Committee, which presents it to Congress, and CMS announces how much it will increase or decrease fees for that year. Meanwhile, a battle is waged in Congress. Each year CMS announces what Congress has set as the adjustment or reduction. Shortly after that, Congress passes a bill that adjusts the fee schedule so that the fees do not decline. Congress passed the "doc-fix" legislation in 2015 eliminating the need to adjust the fee schedule each year. CMS publishes a fee schedule, the Medi-care Physician Fee Schedule (MPFS), for 10,000 physician services.

Until the last few decades, the majority of doctors in this country were in private practice or fee-for-service practice. According to the Bureau of Labor Statistics only 12 percent of physicians were self-employed as of 2009; 19 percent were employed by hospitals; and the remaining 53 percent were paid on a contractual basis and were work-ing in a group practice setting.

Getting back to physicians' income, doctors in private practice must cover office expenses. A doctor needs to employ and pay two and a half (by some counts) staff persons to deal with billing. They spend time obtaining pre-authorization to perform various tests and procedures from insurance companies. Because insurance companies set different limits, the task becomes even more time consuming. According to the AMA, about 20 percent of the claims that insurance companies process are incorrect. All the time doctors spend dealing with paperwork is time that could be spent caring for patients. Time away from patient care also constitutes lost income.[5] It is not surprising to find so many doctors leaving private practice over the last few decades.

Prior to this time, private practice was the standard. Doctors worked hard in the early years of the twentieth century to gain society's respect by embracing a set of practices that they presented as "medical profes-sionalism." Medicine became the model "profession" that many other occupations made every effort to emulate in order to gain some of the privileges that professionalism was providing to doctors, including re-spect, trust, high income, and access to personal information related to illness, and, in the case of MDs, access to the body. The most central feature of medical professionalism was the understanding that the phy-sician would be directly responsible to the patient, rather than to some third party that could stand between the patient and the doctor. This was firmly embedded in the fee-for-service, private practice arrangement. The AMA and its state affiliates were adamant about this. The AMA did not object to medical faculty taking salaried positions because they were primarily engaged in research rather than patient care. So now that an increasing proportion of physicians are accepting salaries—what does that say about medical professionalism?

Indeed, does this mean that they will soon be joining unions to negotiate with the organizations that employ them as a group rather than as individuals?[6] And where does that leave all those other occupations that were so committed to emulating the model of professionalism set forth by physicians? It is worth noting that physicians in private practice, who stood as model professionals for so long, are actually considered small business-persons for legal purposes and are therefore prohibited by law from bargaining collectively, that is, joining unions. Will the shift in employment status change the way they see themselves and their ability to negotiate over wages and benefits with increasingly larger and more powerful health care organizations? It turns out that the topic of professionalism is relevant to the development of nursing as an occupation, to which we turn next.

NURSES

Nursing is the single biggest occupational category in the health sector. According to the National Resources and Services Administration (NRSA), which is part of HHS, there were about 2.8 million nurses in the country in 2013, 62 percent of whom were working in hospitals. Nursing provides an interesting contrast to medicine because it is overwhelmingly a female occupation and because its origins are so different than those of medicine. The history of nursing is heavily influenced by the traditions introduced by Florence Nightingale. Prior to her work during the Crimean War in the 1880s, nursing was not considered a respectable activity for women from good families. It was considered dirty work. Nightingale emphasized the use of skills available to every middle-class young woman, namely, cleaning wounds, changing bandages, and comforting patients. She gained acceptance for nursing as a suitable occupation for a young woman from a respectable family by assuring doctors that nurses were there to assist them, and not get in their way. Therein lay the problem that nursing has faced ever since.

Historically, nursing care was performed by female members of the household largely to care for members of the family who needed such assistance. Only after nursing became an identifiable occupation during the twentieth century did nurses start to work outside the home. Those who worked in the patient's home were called private duty nurses. Their duties were not strictly defined; in addition to nursing care, they ended up doing a little food preparation, a little house cleaning, maybe a little clerical work—whatever the client wanted and the nurse was willing to do.

As hospitals became a more regular source of care during the twentieth century, nurses began doing more work in hospitals. Private duty nursing eventually became defined as less professional. After all, you really didn't have to be a nurse to manage the personal care needs of people who were not acutely ill. As hospitals began caring for more seriously ill patients, nurses needed to have more training.

Nurses' training continued to reflect the philosophy introduced by Florence Nightingale. Nursing schools were opened by hospitals providing something closer to on-the-job training than education with a theoretical base. Nursing students were expected to live in a dorm with strict rules, to be chaperoned, and to perform nursing tasks in the hospital under supervision for three years. Upon graduation they received a diploma and were qualified to take a state licensing exam leading to working as a registered nurse (RN). The relationship between doctors and nurses is best captured by the fact that nurses were expected to stand up when a doctor walked into the room and not sit until the doctor permitted it.

At some point colleges began instituting bachelor's degrees in nursing. After completing four years of college and successfully passing the state licensure exam, a nursing student became an RN, just like the diploma graduate. During the 1960s, when there was so much interest in advancing health care and increasing the pool of health care personnel, two-year associate-degree nursing programs were created. The graduates of those programs also became RNs. This created a problem. There were now three different routes into nursing, based on different levels of education and experience. In other words, nursing, as an occupation, did not establish control over the educational system and entry into the occupation. More troubling was the fact that the content of nursing programs varied across the three entry routes, but the nurses were largely being treated the same way by hospitals, which became their primary employers, no matter which program they completed.

Anytime hospitals faced a shortage of nurses in the past, hospitals did not address the problem by raising nursing salaries, as would happen in most other occupational sectors; they just recruited more student nurses into their diploma programs. Several decades ago, most hospitals closed down their diploma programs as they realized that on-the-job training was not enough to prepare nurses to care for the more seriously ill patients now being admitted to hospitals. This has not benefited nursing as much as one might expect, because hospitals simply began training other kinds of workers to do specific tasks and aggressively recruiting nurses from other countries.

The fact that nursing has traditionally been a female occupation, that nurses have historically been employees rather than independent practitioners like doctors, and that their training does not take nearly as long as medical school are factors that explain nursing's occupational fate up until the last couple of decades or so.

The attention that the effect of nursing care on the health outcomes of hospitalized patients has been receiving over the last few years may alter that perspective. There is a body of evidence developing to indicate that more favorable nurse-to-patient ratios, education, and experience all contribute to better patient outcomes.[7] This together with the unremitting shortage of nurses has brought pressure to bear on legislators. California was the first state to pass a statute requiring hospitals to maintain an eight-to-one patient-to-nursing staff ratio in 2003. The conventional wisdom says that what happens in California predicts what will be happening in other parts of the country in the future. That seems to be true in this case. The battle was successfully waged by the California Nurses Association (CNA), which split off from the American Nurses Association (ANA) because the California nurses wanted to negotiate over wages and working conditions. By 2009, the CNA had joined with National Nurses United, the United American Nurses, and the Massachusetts Nurses Association to form the National Nurses Association (NNA), the largest nurses' union in the country. The ANA continued to say unionism is a threat to the perception of nurses as professionals. However, the success of the NNA is hard to dismiss and the ANA has been forced to give the issue more thought.

One of the steps nursing as an occupation has taken to deal with the problem of professionalism over the last few decades is to carve out niches in which nurses could work more independently. Nursing created a number of "advanced practice" nursing programs, including nurse midwifery (delivering babies), nurse anesthetist programs, and nurse practitioner programs. All of these require master's degree–level training. In addition, there are doctoral-level programs leading to a PhD or doctorate in nursing practice. Nevertheless, doctors are legally authorized to diagnose, prescribe, and treat patients, while nurses are generally not allowed to do so. Some states give broader practice privileges to nurses, meaning that they permit nurse practitioners to have their own offices and their own patients, but even in those instances, doctors have final authority if questions arise.

Like nurse practitioners, certified nurse midwives are considered to be primary health care providers in certain underserved areas. In urban and suburban communities, nurse midwives work with doctors to manage normal pregnancies. Studies regularly show that women are very satisfied with the care they receive from nurse midwives, probably because nurse midwives allow the women more control over the delivery process, allowing them to take more time to deliver. There is no difference in birth outcomes between deliveries managed by nurse midwives and doctors, which may be due to the fact that nurse midwives are willing to refer high-risk pregnancies to doctors. The question this kind of evidence raises is whether greater reliance on such "physician extenders" should be advocated more vigorously.

Nurses with advanced degrees who work in hospitals typically have managerial responsibilities in addition to patient care responsibilities. They oversee the work of licensed practical nurses (LPNs, who receive anywhere from six months to over a year of training), nursing assistants (who receive certification with 160 hours of training), and unit clerks (who are hired without special training to carry out the secretarial tasks for nurses in a hospital).

THERAPISTS

A wide range of occupational groups falls under this designation. Two of the most commonly recognized are physical therapists and occupa-

tional therapists. Activities therapists (in music or art) work with patients who are hospitalized for longer stays. Then there are also less
well-known categories of therapists in hospitals, such as respiratory
therapists. Not all therapists work in hospitals; for example, audiologists
and speech therapists may have private offices and private practices. In
addition, a number of other occupational groups doing psychological
counseling call themselves therapists or counselors. In short, therapists
come to this work from wide-ranging backgrounds and with a variety of
degrees.

TECHNICIANS

Technicians may constitute an even broader category. Medical technicians work in hospital or clinic laboratories. X-ray technicians work
directly with patients and have been around for a long time. There are
now technicians associated with all kinds of new diagnostic equipment
whose work is similar to that of X-ray technicians, for example, sonogra-
phy technicians, mammography technicians, CT technicians, nuclear
medicine technicians, and so on. Many new occupational categories
came on board in hospitals as hospitals created new jobs and trained
people to do particular tasks. For instance, hospitals trained pharmacy
technicians to count pills and bottle them, blood technicians to draw
patients' blood, and so on. Pharmacy technicians are now regularly employed in pharmacies operated by various kinds of stores.

Then there are emergency medicine technicians (EMTs). They attend to people in an ambulance in an emergency situation. Their objective is to stabilize the patient and get him or her to the emergency
room. In some ways their work is comparable to that of physicians'
assistants in the sense that they take direct responsibility for the patient
under the guidance of doctors. In the case of EMTs, they are able to
connect patients to equipment that is monitored by doctors in the
emergency room. But it is the EMTs who administer treatment.

Physicians' assistants (PAs), who don't actually fit neatly into any one
of the designations, perform tasks that a physician assigns to them.
Physicians have been employing increasing numbers of PAs in recent
years. According to the American Association of Physician Assistants, as
of 2008 there were 142 accredited educational programs and 68,124

persons active in the field; over half work in physicians' offices. PAs may also assist in surgery, do continuing care for surgical patients, go on home visits in some parts of the country more than others, and so on. They differ from nurse practitioners in that PAs work under the physician's license, while nurse practitioners work under their own licenses. In other words, the PA may do brain surgery, if the physician who employs him or her is willing to accept responsibility, which is not to say that hospitals would be willing to let this happen. There is a movement to change the name from "physician assistant" to "physician associate," which some physicians agree does more accurately reflect the work of these people.

OTHER PRACTITIONERS

There are two categories of practitioners known as "limited practice" doctors. This includes podiatrists, who are licensed to treat the full range of foot ailments, and dentists, who treat teeth and gums. Dentists and podiatrists are licensed to perform surgery and administer medications. They are doctors. These privileges differentiate them from other practitioners, who may also call themselves doctors. An example is optometrists, who are licensed to examine the eye and prescribe lenses, but must refer patients to an ophthalmologist, who is an MD specializing in the treatment of eye disease, when they detect eye disease.

Similarly, pharmacists are licensed to dispense medications but not prescribe them, even though in many instances they know a great deal more about drug interactions than doctors do. In some hospitals, clinical pharmacists with advanced degrees go on "rounds" together with medical staff to explain drug interactions to medical residents.

ADMINISTRATORS AND OTHER ADMINISTRATIVE WORKERS

Hospital administrators generally come to this work with master's degrees in hospital administration or a comparable degree. The degrees are granted by business schools, schools of public health, medical schools, and a variety of other kinds of programs. The coursework is, however, not all that different. Hospital administrators must be prepared to oversee a wide variety of activities and occupational groups in hospitals and all the other kinds of health care delivery settings (e.g., extended care facilities, outpatient facilities, managed care settings, psychiatric hospitals).

The scope of their responsibility is interesting to consider. Their authority comes from the hospital board of directors or board of trustees, depending on whether the institution is for-profit or nonprofit. They have full authority and responsibility for running the organization on a day-to-day basis. Decisions involving major changes or expenses are the province of the board, and the administrator is responsible for carrying them out. However, one area continues to be somewhat less than clear, although more so in the past than at present: the relationship between hospital administrators and doctors.

One of the biggest responsibilities that falls to administrators is overseeing record keeping. And, as we have seen, there are records of all kinds—the usual ones such as payroll records and purchasing records, of course; more complicated matters revolve around patients' medical files, insurance records, billing records, and anything that might be required in malpractice cases. Protecting the organization from malpractice is a career in and of itself. In fact, a new occupational role called "risk management" came into existence a couple of decades ago. The work of this occupational group is directed to eliminating as many opportunities for malpractice suits as possible—from making sure the railings are sturdy enough to hold up patients who need them, to making sure that patients who want to discuss a problem are put in contact with the person with authority over that area.

Hospital medical records departments, where medical records technicians work, has been one of the fastest-growing areas in the health sector because of the vast amount of information that must be recorded. And it has changed dramatically. Until the last couple of decades of the twentieth century, medical record keeping was a matter of filing pieces of paper. It is now a matter of keeping computerized records and worrying about a whole set of new concerns, especially identifying the right filing code, which determines how much third-party payers will pay the hospital. Representatives of government programs have stepped up efforts to identify and reduce overpayment. With health care reform, if they find that the hospital has been underpaid, it is the hospital's loss. Coding is obviously a matter that attracts the attention of everyone involved in the delivery of health care services.

HEALTH OCCUPATIONS AND HEALTH CARE REFORM

The Affordable Care Act is mandating a number of changes that affect health care occupations. The mandates do not sound extensive when we consider each one separately but when we consider all of them we can see that the cumulative effect turns out to be significant. A few examples of the changes include the Medicare coverage of preventive care services; establishing a nongovernmental agency, the Patient-Centered Outcomes Research Institute (PCORI), a nonprofit agency mandated to track and report clinical effectiveness research results; making five-year demonstration funds available to states to develop alternatives to litigation, that is, tort reform; and allocating funds for training and development of the health care workforce.

The Accountable Care Organizations (ACOs) Rule, which we discussed in the last chapter, has important implications for medical practice. The intent of this initiative is to support the development of "primary care model" medical homes that integrate physical and mental health services and use team management of chronic illness. Doctors were informed that they could set up ACOs without linking up with a hospital, but of course they would then be shouldering all of the risk. A major risk was identified in a joint statement issued by the U.S. Department of Justice (DOJ), the Federal Trade Commission (FTC), and the HHS. The announcement stated that an ACO that grows large enough to provide 50 percent or more of the services in a particular area will come under the scrutiny of these agencies; only those that have 30 percent or less of the market will avoid such scrutiny. In short, physicians, with or without the cooperation of hospitals, are being encouraged to establish these operations but to avoid becoming too successful at it.

QUESTIONS AND ISSUES TO THINK ABOUT

- Is the professionalism that was so central to the identity of physicians in the past being compromised by the fact that they are entering into contracts with large physicians' groups and accepting salaried positions in hospitals? Or does the fact that they have such a high level of knowledge and expertise allow them to redefine what professionalism means these days? Or is professionalism an outdated concept?
- Are doctors' incomes too high? Is there a way to put a cap on how much doctors earn? (We will devote more attention to this in later chapters, but this may be a good time to consider this question. It is something that people mention regularly without giving much thought to how they would like to have doctors' incomes controlled.)
- Nurses are taking bold steps to assert greater control over their work by joining a national union. What is the impact of the issues they are bargaining over on patient care? (You might want to look at the National Nurses Association web site to get a sense of what those issues are.)

5

PRIVATE HEALTH INSURANCE

This is where we finally get to the topic of health insurance coverage, which is at the core of the Affordable Care Act. We begin the chapter with an overview of the origins of health insurance in this country, going on to examine how health insurance has worked over the last eighty years or so. The latter half of the chapter focuses on how the ACA has changed our health care arrangements. The measures the law introduces are exceedingly complicated. However, think of it this way: you will have a better understanding of the law than most Americans and you will be in a position to gloat about that whenever the topic comes up.

Let's begin our assessment of health insurance arrangements by distinguishing between public and private insurance programs. *Public* is code for government-sponsored and supported. *Private* is everything that is not run by the government. Private health insurance comes in two forms: 1) *private, nonprofit* and 2) *private, for-profit*. The difference between nonprofit and for-profit has to do with what happens to the money the organization earns at the end of the year. Just as is true of hospitals and other health care organizations, in for-profit corporations, stockholders, who have invested in the company with the expectation of making money, receive a share of the profits in the form of increased value of the stock they own and, in some cases, payouts called dividends. Nonprofit organizations have no investors and do not earn a "profit." If they take in more than they pay out, the organization puts the "excess" back into the organizational coffers. No individuals get to keep any part of the excess as a bonus. The money is used to upgrade the organization's offerings, equipment, programs, and so forth.

While groups of people here and there may have established funds to help each other in times of need, protection against the costs of health care was not a major concern prior to the 1930s. Two very different models of health insurance coverage came into existence during the first half of the twentieth century—the Blue Cross–Blue Shield (BC-BS) fee-for-service insurance model and the Kaiser Permanente prepaid model. The Great Depression played a role in helping to launch both types of plans. Both were established as nonprofit organizations.

THE FEE-FOR-SERVICE MODEL

The first major insurance plan developed in this country was the Blue Cross plan. It was established by the Baylor University Hospital in Dallas in 1929.[1] The hospital was struggling, like all hospitals during that era, because so many patients could not pay their bills once the Great Depression hit. A review of the records revealed that schoolteachers constituted one clearly identifiable category of people defaulting on their bills. Baylor University Hospital came up with the following plan. It offered the Dallas Board of Education a plan whereby teachers would pay 50 cents a month for twenty-one days of hospital coverage per year. The plan caught on. In fact, it spread across the country. Over the following decade other cities, in many cases whole states, created their own Blue Cross plans, which eventually spawned a Blue Shield addition and became established as BC-BS plans.

The Blue Shield side of the plan evolved more slowly and was initially not nearly as successful as the Blue Cross side. Blue Shield was created to cover physicians' charges. However, it was more difficult to administer because there were so many doctors and so many different services that it was impossible to standardize rates. (Computers have, of course, been programmed to address this problem, not necessarily to solve it.) Also, there was no one to champion this cause. Doctors were not nearly as enthusiastic about instituting insurance arrangements for their services as were hospitals.

The features of the Blue Cross side of the plan were considered groundbreaking at the time. First, it was conceived of as a nonprofit plan, meaning that it was designed to cover its costs and not make a profit. Second, in order to ensure that costs, which were largely unpredictable, would be covered, the people instituting the plan came up with an idea that was considered very innovative. The plan called for everyone to pay the same amount even if they did not have occasion to use any health services. This was called a *community rate*. Whatever the cost was for providing hospital care for everyone in the community (i.e., everyone who signed on for the insurance plan in the region it was operating), plus administrative expenses, determined the *premium* that the enrollees were charged for the coming year. Third, the plan was created by a hospital whose primary concern was covering its costs. Accordingly, Blue Cross paid whatever the hospital charged.

The Blue Cross plan was not designed to monitor hospital costs. Critics have pointed this out, noting that the nature of the plan permitted hospitals to spend as much as they wanted because they could be certain that their expenses would be covered. Blue Cross put no lid on expenditures. Defenders say, that is true, but there were important benefits in this arrangement. By shifting their costs to those who were insured, hospitals could provide care for people who could not afford to be hospitalized. *Cost shifting* became an item on the agenda of public debate during the 1980s. Critics said it was objectionable because it allowed hospitals to be irresponsible about their expenditures and it was unfair to the individuals who were insured but not being hospitalized.

There was nothing underhanded or secret about cost shifting. This was the accustomed method doctors and hospitals used before rates for health care services became standardized. Doctors charged richer patients more than they charged those who had less money. Everyone understood that this was happening. In practicing cost shifting, hospitals were following a well-established pattern. Critics point out that some patients received no care under these conditions if they could not find a doctor and hospital willing to treat them for no money.

When patterns of behavior are followed on a regular basis, sociologists say that the behavior patterns are being institutionalized. One particularly interesting effect of the institutionalized process in this case deserves a little more attention. Because Blue Cross would only pay for hospital care, and not care in the doctor's office, doctors would routinely admit patients to the hospital for tests. Doctors would explain the BC-BS reimbursement arrangements to patients and ask if they would agree to have the necessary tests done in the hospital. The catch was that, officially, Blue Cross would only pay for hospitalization if the patient was sick. Acknowledging this reality, doctors routinely admitted patients with a diagnosis that proved to be negative after the appropriate tests were performed.

Consider the implications of this pattern of behavior. It is less expensive to have tests done on people who walk in, have the test done, and go home. It is much more expensive to keep people in the hospital. Also, as long as the person was going to be there anyway, doctors ordered more tests to justify admitting the person in the first place. Remember that Blue Cross was in the business of reimbursing hospitals for the costs they incurred, so hospitals had no reason to object to this pattern. The hospitals were fully aware of these practices. It was pretty obvious that there were a lot of healthy people being admitted. Doctors were doing it to save their patients money. Patients did not complain about the inconvenience because it did save them money. Both doctors and patients could convince themselves that this was a more efficient way of carrying out tests, that the tests would be more accurate because patients could be monitored before and after the tests, and so on. Eventually, however, health care costs did begin to climb and people did start to complain about it. Now, who is to blame for letting the situation get out of hand? I will leave the answer to that question for you to ponder.

FOR-PROFIT HEALTH INSURANCE

Private, for-profit insurance companies, which sold life insurance, were fairly well established by the 1930s. They exhibited no interest in offering health insurance until Blue Cross developed its plan. The private insurance companies became interested during the early 1940s because demand for health insurance rose rather dramatically around this time. That happened because wages were frozen during World War II and one of the only things that employers could offer to attract workers who were scarce during the wartime period was better benefits, particularly health insurance. Employers discovered that health insurance was particularly attractive to workers. Consider how fast the health insurance business grew—in 1940, only 9 percent of the population had hospital insurance; by 1950 the proportion had risen to 50 percent.[2] Many of the new insurance plans developed during this period were sponsored by privately owned, well-established life insurance companies. The privately owned insurance companies differed from the BC-BS plans in two major ways. First, they operated as *profit-making* rather than *non-profit* enterprises. Second, they reimbursed their enrollees rather than the hospitals in an *indemnity* arrangement (i.e., private insurance companies reimbursed the individual and not the hospital for the costs incurred, meaning the doctor and the hospital billed the patient directly). However, the private companies did not revise the payment schedule used by Blue Cross. Like Blue Cross, they simply paid out whatever hospitals charged. They made sure that they would make a profit by increasing the premium they charged each year, which Blue Cross was doing as well, even if it did not do so to earn a profit. This worked until people started to complain about rising costs.

Insurance companies could have tried to hold down costs much earlier, but no one was pressing them to do that. The economy was booming and health care costs were not rising very fast since insurance plans were far more limited than they are now and few insurance plans covered outpatient care. As the market for health insurance started to become more competitive, the privately owned insurance companies did begin competing based on price. They began setting premiums based on an "experience" or "risk rating" rather than using a "community rating." In other words, they calculated how often particular groups of customers went to the hospital and set the rate accordingly. Furthermore, they began aggressively recruiting customers who would be less likely to run up high health care costs. This has come to be known as "cherry picking" and "cream skimming."

It doesn't take a rocket scientist to figure out that you can attract more business by reducing the premium you charge. The for-profit insurance companies began marketing their plans to organizations employing younger, healthier workers who had safe, quiet office jobs, and, of course, charging less for the offering. When this strategy was initially being developed there were no laws preventing companies from retiring their employees at the age of sixty-five. Insurance companies were not concerned about signing up people who sat all day, probably smoked, and did not get any exercise, because the chances were good that they would not suffer ill health until after they retired (often shortly after they retired) and the company was no longer insuring them. So the private companies succeeded in attracting the younger, healthier employees who were less likely to go into the hospital by charging them less than the BC-BS plans. The BC-BS plans (now more commonly referred to as the "Blues") could not do the same thing because their legal status was that of nonprofit organizations (which meant that they did not have to pay taxes as long as they observed the conditions that made them nonprofits). Accordingly, the Blues could not tailor their rates to particular groups of people. They had to offer a community rate (the same rate for everyone), which was often higher than the experience rate or risk rate (which varied according to the characteristics of the group). Employers, who were becoming more interested in keeping their operating costs down, began offering the less expensive private insurance plans as an alternative to BC-BS.

How would you respond if you were heading up a Blues plan in your region? The only way you can compete with the private insurance companies is to employ the same business practices as they do. In order to offer competitive rates you would have to turn yourself into a profit-making corporation, exactly like the private insurance companies with whom you must compete. Not only did Blues plans turn themselves into for-profit plans, they consolidated their operations through mergers, acquisitions, and joint ventures with for-profit insurers. By 1999, the number of BC-BS plans had fallen from 128 at the peak of expansion to 51.[3] The trend did not let up until the middle of the first decade of the twenty-first century. The number of BC-BS plans is now harder to determine because the companies formed through mergers operate under different names.

THE PREPAID CARE MODEL

It seems that after some small false starts here and there across the country, the idea of prepaid care took root in about 1938 in connection with the construction of the Los Angeles aqueduct. The area was unsettled, with primitive living conditions. Workers were willing to tolerate that, but they were not willing to do dangerous work without some assurance of medical care. No doctor would go to such a setting without some assurances of his own, namely that he could make enough money to set up an office and meet office and living expenses. Henry Kaiser, who headed the company doing the building, hit on a solution. He would guarantee the doctor a predictable income by arranging to have his workers contribute 5 cents per day to assure themselves of the availability of health care services whether they needed care or not. (That meant that the doctor was being paid on what became known as a *capitation* arrangement, not on a fee-for-service basis.) As an aside, Kaiser equipped a train car as a fully outfitted doctor's office that could be moved along as work on the dam progressed. The doctor was saved the money of setting up a permanent office and the workers did not have to travel for care. Pretty innovative, don't you think?

The prepayment arrangement worked so well that Kaiser set up similar programs for his employees during World War II to attract workers to jobs at his shipyards and steel mills in other locations on the West Coast. In 1942, he created a separate organization, Kaiser Permanente, to handle the prepaid health care arrangements for his workers. (The Kaiser Family Foundation is a separate nonprofit organization that carries out health policy–oriented research.) When the war ended, wartime production declined, and employment shifted to other sectors, it looked like Kaiser Permanente would not survive. Henry Kaiser saved the plan by opening it up to the public. And, as they say, the rest is history. Kaiser Permanente evolved into the largest single prepaid care system in the country. As of 2013, it reported having 9.5 million enrollees.

A few other prepaid plans, which stayed local, were established at about the same time as the Kaiser plan. The Health Insurance Plan of Greater New York and the Group Health Cooperative of Puget Sound were two of the largest. Prepaid care arrangements were relatively rare because there was so much opposition to them from the medical establishment (i.e., the AMA and its state and local affiliates). The fee-for-service exchange between the doctor and the patient was one of the traditional, and essential, attributes of medical professionalism, according to the AMA. Consequently, medical societies pressured hospitals to deny admitting privileges (i.e., the right to hospitalize patients) to doctors who were not in a fee-for-service practice. This forced the prepaid plans to build their own hospitals.

Let me repeat, the plans that emerged during the first half of the twentieth century were established as nonprofit entities. The nonprofit

aspect is significant. Remember, this means that there are no share=
holders and no profits to distribute. If earnings exceed projected costs,
the "excess" is plowed back into the organization. That changed mid=
century. This is also when health care costs began to rise, which would
lead to a number of different attempts to hold down costs.

FROM PREPAID CARE TO HEALTH MAINTENANCE

The prepaid care model got an enormous boost from legislation passed
in 1974. This occurred because President Richard Nixon was searching
for a way to put limits on the growth of medical care costs. By this time
it had become clear that the costs of Medicare and Medicaid (estab=
lished in 1965) were running over initial cost projections. Advisors con=
vinced President Nixon that prepaid care was the solution. Advocates
argued that prepaid care would result in savings because the arrange=
ment would encourage people to seek care earlier, before their prob=
lems became more complicated and costly to treat. So, not only was it
going to save money, it would be good for people. President Nixon
presented the plan to the country as something that would help people
maintain their health, which is where the "health maintenance" label
comes from. The medical establishment could not object to this presen=
tation, even though it was firmly opposed to the prepayment feature.
The AMA labeled it "socialized medicine" in a massive media cam=
paign. The AMA's objections notwithstanding, legislation requiring em=
ployers to offer this option to their employees and funding to support
startup costs passed and the term "health maintenance organization," or
HMO, came into widespread use as of that time.

The way this model was designed to work was that both patients and
doctors would sign up with a particular HMO. Doctors would do so by
signing a contract. The earliest HMOs paid doctors a salary; others
offered doctors a contract specifying a fixed amount of money per capi=
ta—a *capitation fee*. There was no restriction on doctors signing up with
more than one HMO. As the HMO model developed, payment ar=
rangements became more complicated. HMOs now often use capita=
tion plus incentives for meeting the organization's budgetary objectives.

Patients would sign on by "enrolling" in a plan that employers had
agreed to offer as a benefit option to employees. The employer would

contract with the HMO to pay a fixed amount of money, the *premium*, to which the employee would contribute a set amount determined by the employer. Patients would be permitted to go only to those doctors who were associated with that particular HMO. HMOs continue to operate under this basic arrangement. Employers who were offering health insurance generally continued to offer fee-for-service insurance options as well.

The fact that the legislation made a considerable amount of money available for startup costs brought many new parties into the prepaid care business, and business turns out to be the right word, too. Initially, the groups that took encouragement from the legislation used Kaiser Permanente as their model. They established themselves as nonprofit organizations. However, it did not take long for that to change. Within a few years, HMOs were being established with the understanding that producing a profit for their owners was exactly what the owners had in mind.

Many of the new HMOs, both for-profit and nonprofit, were established without enough planning, funding, or thought given to administration. Some of the struggling HMOs were bought out. Others simply closed up shop and disappeared. In either case, patients had to sign up with another, possibly new and untested organization, with new doctors, different rules, and so on. This is when the idea that the health care sector was inefficient, lacking in managerial talent, and backward in the application of the latest business techniques took hold. It is also when health sector corporations became more aggressive in their efforts to operate more efficiently in order to gain a greater share of the market, that is, more enrollees.

While the for-profit HMO may not have introduced business practices into the health care sector, it certainly accelerated the application of business practices. The newly evolving HMOs were interested in experimenting with a wide range of business management tools, most notably, monitoring doctors' practice patterns. Collecting and analyzing such information permitted managed care organizations to press doctors to cut the number of patient visits, control the use of expensive tests, and generally reduce expenses associated with treatment.

It took a few more years for HMO executives to realize that one of the main obstacles they faced in trying to control costs or, more importantly, to make a profit, was that the HMOs could only control the costs of patient care taking place within the doctor's office. However, once patients were admitted to the hospital, the HMO lost control. HMOs did have contracts with hospitals covering basic costs per day, but could not really control the additional costs incurred once the patient was admitted. Thus, things like how long a patient was there, what tests were performed, how many times tests were repeated, which all have a big impact on costs, were not under the control of the HMO. They needed to gain more control over the hospital and thus over every other stage of care. That meant managing the care of the patient at all stages of treatment. This is what brought us to the next iteration in the labeling process—the era of *managed care*. Managing patient care led to managing the organizations and all the personnel patients interact with.

Here we move into how economists explain the operations of private sector organizations. As HMOs became larger and more powerful, they were able to demand better deals in negotiations with hospitals and all the companies from which they order equipment and supplies (economies of scale). In many cases, managed care organizations could and ultimately did simply buy out their suppliers (vertical integration). This created even larger and more powerful organizations. Business executives argued that it was self-evident that "competition is healthy!" And that explains how we moved from the HMO label to the *managed competition* label. Managed competition was the foundational idea on which the Clinton health care reform plan was based. The managed competition concept was tainted by the failure of the Clinton health care reform proposal and fell into disfavor. Health insurance companies announced that they would prefer their offerings to be known as "health care plans."

As to personnel, it is worth noting that the Kaiser Permanente plan was established with the aim of providing both continuing and preventive care by relying more heavily on care provided by generalists or primary care practitioners (PCPs), as opposed to specialists or surgeons. The newly established HMOs adopted this strategy as well. Internists, pediatricians, and family practitioners, the PCPs, were expected to act as gatekeepers. They were expected to accept responsibility for treating most of the patient's problems—referring patients to a specialist only if a problem truly required considerably more specialized knowledge. By monitoring the patient's care more closely, gatekeepers were to keep patients out of the hospital, which is beneficial to the patient (unless, of course, that effort becomes too restrictive). Hospitalization is the main form of care that HMOs intentionally tried to restrict because it is so much more expensive than care provided in the doctor's office. For their part, the primary care doctors began to complain that the HMOs were imposing too many restrictions on what they could do, pressuring them to see more patients than they could handle, imposing time limits on patient visits, and so on.

As an aside, the provision of preventive and continuing care is the way the ACA expects Accountable Care Organizations to work. The rapid growth in the number of ACOs indicates that both doctors and hospitals have embraced this approach. While the prepaid care label is generally not used to describe ACOs, the managed care label is used but sparingly. "Medical home" is the new label used to describe how ACOs are meant to operate.

Curiously, even though employers had seen little evidence that managed care was reducing costs during the 1980s, they suddenly became convinced that managed care was the way to go during the 1990s. Employers began dropping traditional insurance as an alternative in the health care benefit packages they were offering to employees. In 1993, roughly half of American workers (versus the population as a whole) were enrolled in managed care programs; by 1995, that figure leaped to 73 percent).[4] The speed of the shift surprised everyone. While arguments about the pros and cons of managed care continued to mount, the number of people enrolled in health maintenance plans increased steadily through the decade of the 1990s. Enrollment peaked in 1999 at 30.1 million but has been declining since then.[5]

Enrollees, that is, patients, began expressing a rising level of dissatisfaction with the HMO model during the late 1980s and early 1990s. While they were unhappy about the rising costs, they were registering most dissatisfaction about the restrictions imposed by HMOs, especially on which doctors they could see and how long they could stay in the hospital—being discharged "quicker and sicker." By 1996, twenty-nine states had passed laws governing early discharge. The rising level of dissatisfaction led to the introduction of a variation known as the "preferred provider organization," or PPO. The PPO option allowed enrollees to pay a higher premium for the right to select doctors of their own choosing. When that adjustment did not seem to fully overcome enrollee dissatisfaction, a "point-of-service" (POS) option appeared. This required the enrollee to select a primary care physician from the approved list, now known as a network, who would assume responsibility for recommending a specialist if necessary. The POS was offered at a higher premium than the HMO premium, but one that was lower than the PPO option.

The most recent creation is the EPO, which stands for Exclusive Provider Organization. It is like an HMO in that care outside of the network is not covered. However, EPOs may permit enrollees to refer themselves to a specialist within the network.

Critics were quick to point out that the alternative arrangements were giving employers an excuse to revise benefit plans and pass on a greater proportion of the premium to employees. Health plans took the opportunity to promote the PPO, POS, and EPO as innovations rising out of the preferences consumers were registering, that is, presenting it all as the new era of "consumer-driven health care."

One of the other options health plans had been promoting in recent years as part of the consumer-driven health care arrangements is the *high deductible plan* option accompanied by a health savings account. Such plans had a lower premium because insurance coverage would start after the enrollee spent a substantial amount of money out of his or her own pocket; depending on the plan this could be $1,000, $2,000, $5,000, or more. This is the deductible. To make the high deductible option more attractive, legislation passed in 2003 created health savings accounts (HSAs). The HSA allowed the enrollee to set aside a certain amount of income in a tax-free account to be used to cover medical costs that fell in the deductible range. According to a 2008 study by the Government Accountability Office (GAO), the average income of those who opted for the HSA plan was $139,000, compared to the income of average enrollees, which was $57,000. Critics pointed out that this amounted to another tax loophole that was advantageous to the rich and was not something that benefited most Americans.

That brings us to a rather basic question, namely, whether the business approach employed by health insurance companies was in fact resulting in increased efficiency and was the best way to control rising costs. In assessing whether the business approach was succeeding, it is important to understand that the primary objective of for-profit health plans is making money, it is their "legal, ethical, and fiduciary responsibility" to do so.[6] Accordingly, the industry as a whole refers to the money spent on medical care as the "medical-*loss* ratio." The money spent on medical care carries a negative label because of its negative impact on the bottom line. The logic that flows from the use of that concept is obvious—cut medical care services in order to increase profits. Critics of the business approach say that consolidation, one of the main mechanisms the industry was using, is less a matter of efficiency than an attempt to increase control over the market. (There is a great deal more to say about the pros and cons associated with the business approach to health care delivery, which we will address in chapter 9.)

The five largest health insurance companies got to where they are because of numerous previous mergers. This is when the Federal Trade Commission (FTC) and states' attorneys started to take an interest, because the number of insurers had clearly been declining. The FTC's concern was that certain mergers would produce organizations so large that their size would result in restraint of trade, meaning that they would be the major and perhaps only insurer in the area. States' attorneys were concerned because enrollees in their states would have little choice in selecting an insurance plan and there would be no competition to keep the cost of insurance in check. Policy makers and, more to the point, the courts were weighing this question: are health plan mergers helping to contain costs or does consolidation of such magnitude create monopolies with the power to set prices for the purpose of enhancing profit with no real interest in containing costs? The upshot of that was the creation of the U.S. Department of Justice and Federal Trade Commission Horizontal Merger Guidelines in 1997. ("Market concentration" is another topic to which we will return in chapter 9.)

Another criticism of health insurance companies that surfaces periodically focuses on the compensation awarded to company executives. This criticism was voiced more often during the early years of the twenty-first century before attention switched rather decisively to debates about the pros and cons of health care reform. Critics were readier to point out that the health plan executives were getting rich by denying care to people who are sick. A case in point was the 2003 package that went to Aetna's CEO, John Rowe.[7] While his compensation package is not atypical, there was a special twist in his case. He received $1,042,146 in salary, a $2.2 million bonus, new stock options that were estimated to be worth $5.6 million, and a $7 million cash payment on stock options, plus other compensation of nearly $400,000. That is a staggering $16,242,146 in total. Other officers of the company received huge compensation packages as well that year. One group of investors decided to take action. The United Association of Plumbers, Pipefitters & Sprinklerfitters proposed to shareholders and the board of directors of Aetna that Rowe's compensation package be limited to $1 million and annual bonuses be linked to performance measures. The board rejected the proposal, saying that it was too rigid. The union's move was spurred on by the company's decision to fire 10,700 employees and lay off an additional 700 over the previous year.

Attention to compensation going to health insurance company CEOs, as well as CEOs in other sectors, has been attracting greater attention lately as concern about increasing inequality is registered by various observers, including the rich who are not in the top 1 percent. CEOs are benefiting from the rise in the value of company stock. According to one report, "Profits at the nation's seven largest publicly traded insurers went up in 2010 as plans spent less on care and used income to buy back their stock to boost per-share earnings."[8]

Some observers pointed out that health insurance companies expected greater profits once the ACA was fully implemented because of increased enrollments. In expectation of the restrictions and oversight that the ACA would impose, insurance companies took steps to increase premiums. When such moves hit the media, the companies being mentioned did reduce their rates.

There are also those who were arguing that health insurance companies were making a modest profit compared to some other industries. Some estimates put profits at 3 to 4 percent. This is in contrast to what the business pages told us was the most profitable industry in the United States at the time, that is, mining and crude oil extraction, which reported just under 20 percent in annual profits in 2009. More closely related to this discussion, would you be surprised to discover that the pharmaceutical industry was the second most profitable industry, reporting a return of 19.8 percent in 2009? This caused some health policy makers to ask: How much profit is reasonable when we are dealing with people's pain and suffering? How much profit are pharmaceutical companies making on life-saving medications? How much should we be spending on medications that people don't really need but are being convinced will perform miracles by the constant barrage of ads? (More on this in chapter 9.)

COVERAGE AND COST OF WORKPLACE HEALTH INSURANCE

Let's take a closer look at how many people receive health insurance through their employers and then consider the plight of those who are not receiving this benefit. As costs began to escalate, employers initially tried to cut their costs by switching to less expensive plans and limiting the number of plans employees could choose from. However, this did little to cap the steady rise in costs. Over time, private sector employers (as opposed to public sector employers) began dropping the health insurance benefit. In 2000, 69.7 percent were covered by employer-sponsored health insurance; by 2011 that figure dropped to 59.5 percent; the figure is even lower for employees between the ages of eighteen and sixty-five, at 52.4 percent.[9] Part of the explanation for the decline is that fewer employees were signing on to the insurance employers were offering because the employees' share had become so expensive. There are no rules on how much of the share of the cost of insurance employers can require employees to pay. So how much has the employees' share risen? The average annual premium for an individual employee's share increased from $2,490 in 2000 to $5,384 in 2012; for family coverage it went from $6,415 to $15,473. That is before additional costs of actually using health care services, including copay for each visit or prescription and deductibles at the beginning of each year. (As you will recall, these concepts came up in chapter 2 in conjunction with the Kaiser quiz on definitions. We will also discuss them in more detail in the next chapter.) Doesn't that go a long way in explaining why so many people have been saying that something has to be done about the cost of health care?

THE INDIVIDUAL HEALTH INSURANCE MARKET

That brings us to the question of what one could do if one's employer decided to drop health insurance as a benefit, if the share the company expected employees to pay became too high, one was either self-employed or unemployed, or working for a small company that had never offered health insurance benefits. Why couldn't one just go out and buy an individual health insurance policy, recognizing that it would probably be somewhat more expensive than getting insurance through an employer?

A small proportion of the population had been obtaining health insurance on an individual basis in the individual health insurance market prior to the passage of the ACA. In 2009, 5.3 percent of the population had individual health insurance.[10] Why more people weren't buying their own health insurance is not hard to explain. There are two basic reasons. One, they couldn't afford it; and, two, insurance companies would not sell it to them. Prior to 2010 insurance companies were under no obligation to sell insurance to everyone who applied for it. From the perspective of insurance companies, enrolling individuals is much riskier than enrolling a large number of employees working for a single company. Enrolling individuals who have a pre-existing health problem is especially risky. Why accept such risk if you don't have to?

Consider the story told by a woman who tried to get insurance before passage of the ACA. She found herself without insurance when her company was bought out and she lost her job. Her husband was retired so he did not have a policy that would provide insurance coverage for her.

> My husband, teenage daughter and I were all active and healthy, and naively thought getting health insurance would be simple. . . . First, we wanted to know that, if we had a medical catastrophe, we would not exhaust our savings. Second, uninsured patients are billed more than the rates that insurers negotiate with doctors and hospitals, and we wanted to pay those lower rates. The difference is significant: my recent MRI cost $1,300 at the "retail" rate, while the rate negotiated by the insurance company was $700. . . . I diligently listed the various minor complaints for which we had been seen over the years, knowing that these might turn up later and be a basis for revoking coverage if they were not disclosed.
>
> Then the first letter arrived—denied. . . . Why were we denied? What were these preexisting conditions that put us into high-risk categories? For me, it was a corn on my toe for which my podiatrist had recommended an in-office procedure. My daughter was denied because she takes a regular medication for a common teenage issue. My husband was denied because his ophthalmologist had identified a slow-growing cataract. . . .
>
> I completed four applications for each of the three of us, using reams of paper. I learned to read the questions carefully. I mulled

over the difference between a "condition" and "something for which you have sought treatment." I was precise and succinct. I felt as if was doing a deposition.[11]

She goes on to say that she was not able to obtain a family policy but was able to obtain individual health insurance policies for each of them. Their individual premiums increased substantially over the following six years, with an average increase of 20 percent per year.

The economic recession (remember this was the biggest recession since the Great Depression of 1929) that we experienced during the first decade of the twenty-first century caused the ranks of the unemployed to swell. A study carried out by the Commonwealth Fund found that of the 3,033 persons surveyed nearly one-quarter lost their jobs between 2008 and 2010. Extrapolating that, about 43 million people lost their jobs. "Of the estimated 26 million adults who bought, or tried to buy, health insurance on the individual insurance market during that period, 16 million found it very difficult or impossible to find a plan they could afford. An estimated 9 million were turned down or charged a higher price because of a health problem, or a preexisting condition that excluded them from their coverage."[12]

Okay, so you couldn't get insurance for all the reasons just mentioned. What didn't people just pay for their health care until they did get insured? The main problem is that as an individual, a person has no bargaining power. Most of us would go to the hospital and have an essential or life-saving surgical procedure done without weighing the costs and benefits, right? Then people get the bill. The bill turns out to be a lot higher than the bill insured people were issued for the same procedure. Uninsured persons were being billed at the full (whatever the hospital wanted to charge) rate set by the hospital and not the rate the insurance company established through a contract with the hospital. If the person without insurance coverage was charged the non-negotiated amount, couldn't the person negotiate after the fact? Maybe. Could that person afford to pay the renegotiated charge—maybe, maybe not. And, that explains why so many people were going into medical bankruptcy. About one-half the bankruptcies in this country over recent years have been attributed to medical debt.

Legislation has been in place since 1986 requiring insurance companies to provide continued coverage for a certain period of time after the employee leaves his or her place of employment. This is known as COBRA (passed under the Consolidated Omnibus Budget Reconciliation Act of 1986). The legislation does not address costs. Insurance companies can charge whatever they want for continued coverage. As a result, people who suddenly found themselves unemployed were entitled to receive that coverage, but might not have been able to afford it.

Now that you understand how health insurance was working prior to 2010, let's look at how the ACA changed things. As you know, according to some it is a move in the right direction and according to others it is a major disaster and should be abolished. In order to enter into that debate, understanding what the ACA has introduced is essential—not that this part of the discussion is easy to comprehend. But dividing it into two basic parts should help: the individual mandate and the employer mandate.

HEALTH CARE REFORM: THE INDIVIDUAL MANDATE

The individual mandate is one of the most controversial parts of the health care reform law. The law required every individual in the country, with some limited and very clearly identified exceptions, to have health insurance as of 2014. Fines are imposed on everyone who does not obtain coverage to be collected as part of the tax return for the following year. The amount of the fine was to be phased in: at $95 per person in 2014 or 1 percent of taxable income, whichever is higher; $325 in 2015 or 2 percent of taxable income; $695 or 2.5 percent of taxable income up to a maximum of $2,085 per family income as of 2016. After 2016, the fine increases annually by the cost-of-living adjustment. Exceptions to this are allowed for a limited number of reasons, including financial hardship, religious objections, for persons without coverage for less than three months, incarcerated persons, undocumented immigrants, and American Indians. An exception is also made for those whose incomes fall below the tax filing threshold and those who are unable to find a plan that costs less than 8 percent of their income. Everyone earning 133 percent of the federal poverty level or less was to be eligible for Medicaid coverage as of 2014. (We will discuss the Medicaid program in chapter 6.) This did not happen. The explanation has to do with Health Exchanges, to which we will get shortly.

The rationale for requiring all individuals to purchase health insurance is that it prevents people from buying insurance only when they need it. As some pundits put it, deciding to buy it on the way to the hospital. Allowing people to avoid paying until they need health care is obviously not fair to all those who paid in all along. Having healthy people as well as sick people in the insurance pool spreads the risk. As you will recall this is the basis on which both the BC-BS and the Kaiser Permanente plans were founded. And the basis on which private insurance operates when it lowers costs to companies that employ persons who are estimated to pose a lower risk.

To ensure that individuals have a range of insurance plans from which to choose, states were mandated to establish *Health Exchanges,* which would operate as health insurance marketplaces. The intent was to allow people to shop for insurance policies. In fact, the exchanges are now being referred to as *marketplaces.* They carry different names in each state.

In order to ensure that states would in fact create health exchanges, the ACA stipulated that states would lose the federal funding supporting the state Medicaid program if they did not do two things. First, expand Medicaid to cover all or nearly all poor people in the state; and, second, set up a state Health Exchange to be used by all those who were not currently insured but required to buy an insurance policy. The federal government distributed $4 billion in start-up funds for this purpose. Funding was available up to January 2015. According to a December 5, 2014, report in *Crain's Chicago Business,* states that did not set up exchanges "left the money on the table," which in the case of Illinois was about $270 million. (This is another point to which we will return in chapter 9.)

Since Medicaid is one of the most costly budget items in most states, refusing to set up an Exchange would result in very serious financial loss. The law also made clear that the federal government would step in and create a federally facilitated Health Exchange in such a case. However, in 2012 the Supreme Court found the Medicaid expansion section of the ACA to be unconstitutional. The decision meant that the state would be able to keep the Medicaid funds it was already receiving without expanding its Medicaid program. The ruling effectively eliminated the requirement that states create a Health Exchange since states would suffer no penalty for refusing to do so. As of 2015 the breakdown in choices made by states is as follows: fourteen state-based Exchanges; ten state partnerships or federally supported partnerships; twenty-seven federally facilitated. Because the administration had not expected that it would need to create so many federally facilitated Exchanges, the federally sponsored web site was unable to deal with so many enrollees at one time. That resulted in the disastrous "rollout" in 2013, the first year during which enrollment was required.

The new contractor hired to fix the web site succeeded in making it work in time for the second enrollment period. Commenting on the initial rollout, a number of high-tech consultants said that glitches are not unusual in launching new web sites, noting such things get worked out, are quickly forgotten, and have little impact on the products being launched. The fact that the second rollout received little media attention supports those observations.

THE HEALTH MARKETPLACE

States were given the authority to determine which insurance companies can participate in the state's Exchange. The ACA does require companies to meet certain qualifications. They must have adequate provider networks, be accredited, perform well with respect to quality measures, and so on. They must agree to report information on claims payments, enrollment and disenrollment, number of claims denied, cost sharing, and so on. Insurance companies are allowed to "risk rate," to a limited extent. They may charge some people more, on the basis of age, but no more than three times more from youngest to oldest enrollees. They may also have higher premiums for smokers.

As an aside, it did not take long for this stipulation to present problems. The rationale for instituting a smoking disincentive was clear. There was little disagreement. However, more recently policy analysts have reversed their position, pointing out that smokers disproportionately fall into a lower income category. Assessing a higher premium could mean that many would not be able to afford the insurance. Since smokers are at higher risk of illness, being shut out of the health care system could very well increase the cost of their care, which would increase national health care costs. Some states have already dropped this stipulation. Interesting, isn't it, to see unexpected insights altering what initially looked to be well thought out regulations?

The feature that people shopping for health insurance were expected to appreciate most is the requirement that insurance companies state what they cover in plain language so that potential enrollees can compare plans using the same criteria. Highly desirable, yes. Doable, not so much. Other rules include the following: insurers are prohibited from using preexisting health conditions in setting rates; imposing lifetime limits on coverage; and rescinding coverage except in cases of fraud. They are required to present plans to increase premiums for review and limit waiting periods for coverage to ninety days. One of the most popular changes permits young adults to stay on their parents' health plans until age twenty-six.

The most clearly defined mandate issued by the ACA is the requirement that insurance companies offer plans that fall into one of four benefit categories plus one catastrophic category. They are not required to offer plans in all four categories.

- Bronze plan—provides basic coverage; those who purchase this plan are responsible for paying for 40 percent of costs of care out of their own pockets. (Limits on out-of-pocket costs are linked to income. The bronze plan has the lowest premium, that is, the purchase price, because it allows for the highest out-of-pocket costs. The premiums increase in the other three plans and the out-of-pocket costs decrease.)
- Silver plan—provides basic coverage with 30 percent out-of-pocket costs
- Gold plan—enrollees pay 20 percent out-of-pocket
- Platinum plan—enrollees pay 10 percent out-of-pocket
- Catastrophic plan—available to persons thirty years and younger; covers three primary care visits; all else is out-of-pocket but with a defined maximum figure for total costs.

Tax benefits are available to persons with incomes up to 400 percent of poverty. (The government calculates and reports poverty guidelines on an annual basis.) The law permits enrollees to use the tax benefit to reduce the cost of the monthly premium or as a tax rebate at the end of the tax year. Insurance subsidies are available to persons whose earnings fall under 250 percent of poverty. Subsidies are to cover copayments, deductibles, and coinsurance. (The specific numbers involved are posted on the CMS site.)

It is not surprising then that many people were confused about all of this, not sure whether they were entitled to tax benefits and tax subsidies, not sure where to get information and help interpreting it, and not sure how to go about it all. The requirement that insurance companies make their plans clear did not overcome the fact that insurance companies were offering multiple plans within each of the four categories. The number of plans can run into the hundreds. Comparing them all is obviously not easy. The solution to the complexities involved in choosing a plan turned out to be "navigators." The government made funds available to states to train people to serve as helpers, now often called "health advocates." They are there to help people navigate the health insurance marketplace. A larger number of navigators were trained to help during the second enrollment year in 2014.

CHANGES TO PRIVATE INSURANCE PLANS

The ACA requires health insurance plans to report the proportion of premium dollars they spend on clinical services. Those that spent less than 85 percent on services were mandated to provide rebates to enrollees as of January 1, 2011. As you will recall, the insurance industry label for the remaining 15 percent is *medical-loss ratio*. The law prohibits insurance plans from spending more than 15 percent on anything other than health care services, that is, administration, salaries, benefits, and distribution of profits. In the individual and small group market, the medical-loss ratio cap was set at 20 percent.

HEALTH CARE REFORM: THE EMPLOYER MANDATE

The law requires employers with 200 employees or more to enroll all full-time employees, defined as those working thirty hours or more, in a plan or plans selected by the employer. The prediction was that this would cause companies to move more employees into part-time positions to avoid providing insurance. There is little evidence to indicate that this has happened to a noticeable extent. The legislation has minimal effect on the large companies that have been providing health insurance for their employees all along.

The law imposed a fine of $2,000 on all employers with fifty or more employees who did not provide coverage as of 2014. The effect of this on small employers turned out to be just as controversial as the individual mandate. As a result the Small Employer mandate was delayed until 2015 and again until 2016. The revised deadline became even more complicated. Employers with one hundred plus employees were required to cover 70 percent of their employees by 2015 and 95 percent by 2016.

Employers who have fewer than fifty employees were encouraged to provide insurance but not required to do so. It is important to recognize that 96 percent of companies have fewer than fifty employees, which means that the vast majority of employers are not affected by the ACA.

The law requires states to create Small Business Health Options Program (SHOP) Exchanges as of 2017 in order to help small businesses purchase coverage. Why small companies have been reluctant to provide insurance, according to the Small Business Administration, is that on average, they have been paying 18 percent more than larger companies. Employers with ten or fewer employees whose annual wages average out to $25,000 or less are eligible for a full tax credit for providing insurance.

QUESTIONS AND ISSUES TO THINK ABOUT

- Opponents of the ACA have been arguing for the elimination of the individual mandate to be replaced by Health Savings Accounts (HSAs). They say that the tax-free feature of HSAs would allow Americans to put aside money for the specific purpose of buying health insurance. This would, in turn, give people a greater choice in the amount they want to save and the price they want to pay for an insurance policy. What do you think of this alternative?
- This is a tough one. Is allowing insurance companies to charge smokers a higher premium a good idea or not considering that more poor

people smoke and the higher charge might prevent them from being able to afford to purchase health insurance?

- A few large corporations have announced that they plan to pay the penalty and not insure their employees because the penalty ($2,000 per employee in 2014) would cost them less than paying their share of an employee health insurance policy. Some employers have said that they would also give their employees an additional amount of money to help them pay for their own insurance. (It is not clear how many employers have actually done any of this.) Taking the role of a health policy maker, would you argue that there would be an advantage to allowing companies to pay the penalty and give their employees a certain amount of money to buy their own insurance? Are there any variations on this approach that you would be willing to support?

6

PUBLIC HEALTH INSURANCE

The federal government created three government-sponsored, that is, public, health insurance programs during the last half century: Medicare, the program for the elderly; Medicaid, the program for the poor; and the State Children's Health Insurance Program (CHIP) for low-income children. The government also operates programs that provide health care services for some other clearly specified categories of persons. This includes the Veterans Administration (VA) for veterans, Federal Employees (FEHB), military personnel (TRICARE), and the Indian Health Service (IHS) for Native Americans.

Medicare and social security are considered "entitlement" programs, programs that people are entitled to. As we saw in chapter 2 in examining the origins of social security, the benefits that come with social security were defined as something that people earned over their lifetime by working and contributing to the program. The same definition applies to the Medicare program. This is in contrast to programs for which people qualify because they don't have the "means" to purchase the services they need—these are known as "means tested" programs. Medicaid and CHIP are means-tested programs.

The programs are complicated. I leave it to you to decide whether they are more complicated than the private insurance plans we have just looked at. If you end up feeling overwhelmed by how much you need to know about the plans, you can appreciate how everyone who is trying to enroll in a health insurance plan feels. And just imagine how older people, who may not be so comfortable with obtaining information found on Internet sites, must feel.

MEDICARE

The Medicare program was legislated in 1965 as an amendment (Title 18) to the Social Security Act. It went into operation in July 1966; the first full year of operation was 1967. It was designed to provide health insurance for people over the age of sixty-five. As you will recall from an earlier discussion, this was done because the elderly were identified as particularly vulnerable at that time. They were found to be at greater risk of not having the resources to pay for health care and at greater risk of experiencing illness. The focus on poverty in the early 1960s led to the discovery that an unexpectedly high proportion of older Americans were poor. Making things more complicated, not only were poor Americans unable to afford to buy their own health insurance after retirement, it was not readily available on an individual basis, especially not to people over the age of sixty-five.

Most Americans become eligible for Medicare once they reach the age of sixty-five. Younger persons who are permanently disabled or blind may qualify as well. Persons with end-stage renal disease (meaning it is fatal unless the person has a kidney transplant) were included in 1972 because someone in Congress advocated for it and no one particularly objected.

The plan is complex. But the enrollment process is easy—all a person has to do is call Social Security and give one's name to a real person. The following describes the plan before the changes outlined in the ACA reform act went into effect. The enrollment and expenditure data are based on the most recent reports. Medicare was originally established as a two-part program: Part A is the hospital insurance portion and Part B covers physicians' fees. Two newer parts, labeled Parts C and D, were added later. Part C, which is now known as Medicare-Advantage, is an option that allows people to join Medicare-approved, alternative plans offered by private insurance companies that combine Parts A and B and sometimes include Part D. Part D is the prescription drug plan legislated in 2003.

Anyone who has paid into the social security fund or Railroad Retirement Board for ten years or more is automatically eligible for Part A. Part B covers doctors' services, is voluntary, and carries a monthly charge, which is deducted from the person's monthly social security check. A person must sign up for Part B once the person is eligible for social security benefits. Medicare enrollees may choose to purchase C and D plans from private insurance companies. The government outlines all the components of the Medicare plan in a manual that is updated every year and sent out to all enrollees and made available on its web site as well. The amount of detail is overwhelming. I will provide an overview rather than trying to include all the special conditions, exceptions, and variations.

As of 2014, Medicare enrolled 55 million persons with a budget of $605.9 billion. That makes it the most expensive of the three public health programs but not the largest in terms of enrollment. These figures also raise concerns about sustainability, which we will address later in this discussion.

Part A is funded through the 1.45 percent payroll deduction plus a 1.45 percent contribution on the part of the employer over the person's entire work history. Part A also covers skilled nursing home care, but sets strict limitations. Nursing home coverage is available for one hundred days, but only after three or more days of hospitalization. There is no copayment for the first twenty days, meaning that Medicare covers the entire cost. There is a daily charge after twenty-one days. Medicare pays nothing after one hundred days.

Part B is funded through a deduction in the enrollee's social security check (not payroll check). People must sign up for it and pay on a monthly basis. In addition to the monthly premium, enrollees pay an annual deductible (this is a one-time-only amount) plus coinsurance, which is generally 20 percent of all Medicare-approved doctor and outpatient charges.

The Medicare plan does not cover a number of things that you might expect it to cover, like long-term nursing home care after one hundred days, as just mentioned. Since there are a lot of people in nursing homes—who is paying for their care? It turns out that Medicaid is probably paying. We will get back to that. Medicare does not pay for dental care, hearing aids, and hearing exams, routine eye care and most eyeglasses, or such necessities as adult diapers. (Before you question these restrictions, where would you suggest the money for those things come from? You might want to go back a couple of paragraphs and notice how much Medicare is already spending. All of it coming from tax dollars. Medicaid does pay for most of these things.)

Because coinsurance and deductibles can run into a lot of money, Medigap insurance was created. As of 2015, there are ten standardized Medigap plans (the number has varied from year to year as some were discontinued); they can be sold by any private insurance company that wishes to offer one or more of them, as long as the plan covers whatever is specified by the government in the ten plans identified by some of the letters running A through N. The government publishes a booklet in hard-copy and online versions outlining what the plans identified by each letter are supposed to cover. Companies are permitted to set the prices they charge and claim that they provide better administrative services. They cannot claim that they will provide more health care services than specified by the plan under that letter. This was done in the effort to eliminate what we think of as the "fine print."

Part C was known as Medicare + Choice when it was introduced in 1997. Under this arrangement, Medicare was to pay private insurance companies a fixed fee to provide a package of health care services, combining Parts A and B. The number of plans grew to 345 by the following year. When the government looked into who was choosing to enroll in Medicare + Choice plans, it discovered that enrollees were generally younger and healthier than the general Medicare population. Moreover, it found that those who did become seriously ill proceeded to drop out of these plans and shift back to the traditional Medicare plan. Given these findings, Medicare determined that it was overpaying and proceeded to reduce the rate that it was offering private insurance companies to provide alternative plans. Medicare + Choice plans responded by increasing their out-of-pocket charges. By 1999, 17 percent of the Medicare-eligible population opted for this alternative. The out-of-pocket charges averaged $429 that year. The charges rose steadily after that. By 2003 charges stood at $1,260 per year. By 2004 the number of plans had dropped to 145 and the number of enrollees had dropped to 11 percent.[1] Since then enrollment has been rising steadily and stood at about 30 percent as of 2014.

The rules governing Medicare + Choice were revised in 2003 in conjunction with the passage of Part D, the Medicare Prescription

Drug, Improvement, and Modernization Act. The Part C part of the plan was renamed Medicare Advantage. In passing this legislation the government agreed to pay insurance companies 8.4 percent more per Medicare Advantage enrollee than for enrollees in the Part A and B traditional plan. Proponents presented it as a cost containment measure. The members of Congress who presented this argument said that private companies needed an incentive to offer alternatives to government plans, which would ultimately reduce costs through competition because private companies were sure to introduce cost-saving innovation. By all accounts, over the next few years the amount the government was paying private companies over and above the cost of Part A and Part B edged up to 14 percent, reaching a high of 19 percent in some rural areas.[2]

That brings us to Part D, the prescription drug legislation, the Medicare Prescription Drug, Improvement, and Modernization Act, signed into law in 2003 at a cost of $395 billion. Two months later, the White House announced that it had recalculated that figure and found that it would actually cost $534 billion.[3] Unfortunately, this came at a time when the costs of the war in Iraq were running higher than predicted and the economy was not improving as fast as the White House had said it would.

Part D went into effect in 2006. It was designed to be offered by private insurance companies. Medicare enrollees could select from a range of plans offered by private companies and sign up on a voluntary basis. The unique feature of the plan, the *doughnut hole*, was the result of the compromise that Congress reached because there was not enough money to provide for full coverage. During its first year of operation it worked as follows: the plan covered 75 percent of drug costs up to $2,250. After that, the person would pay 100 percent for drugs—putting the person in the doughnut hole. After a person spent $5,100, coverage would kick back in again to cover 95 percent of the cost of drugs. Expenditures between $2,250 and $5,100 defined the doughnut hole. The doughnut hole was scheduled to change in size with every passing year, as was the percentage of costs covered beyond the doughnut hole. As of 2011, enrollees were covered at the rate of 75 percent for expenditures up to $2,840; zero until $6,448, when coverage at the rate of 80 percent kicked in again. However, because many more drugs were now being offered as generics rather than patented drugs, cost had dropped considerably.

Part D plans are sold by insurance companies on a state-by-state basis. The number of plans enrollees may choose from averages around thirty or thirty-five per state out of a total of 1,001. As of 2015, plans were being sold at a range of premiums, from a low of $14.80 per month to a high of around $45.00. The rules for which drugs are covered and at what rate are complicated depending on whether the drugs are generic formulations and on a variety of other rules over which the government has little say. The law that created Medicare specifically prohibits it from engaging in any bargaining over the price of pharmaceuticals or the prices charged by the Part D insurance plans. The doughnut hole compromise resulted from the fact that 73 percent of the cost of Part D is financed through general tax revenues.[4]

Administration

The Medicare program is administered by the CMS, which is part of HHS. CMS does not employ staff to process Medicare claims. It enters into contracts with insurance companies, known as Medicare Administrative Contractors (MACs), who compete for the contracts. They are paid to carry out the day-to-day administration of the program. They do the paperwork and pay the bills submitted by hospitals and doctors.

CMS also monitors the quality of the care for which it is paying. As you will recall from chapters 4 and 5, CMS requires that hospitals be accredited by the Joint Commission, the organization that reviews the performance of hospitals in the United States. The CMS does its own reviews as well. It monitors doctors' performance by contracting with peer review organizations (PROs). Doctors perform the peer review, the idea being that you need to be a doctor to evaluate whether other doctors are doing a good job. The PROs employ a staff of workers, usually nurses, who review Medicare files for the purpose of finding unusual patterns of treatment or charges. When there is some question about treatment, doctors who work with the PRO become involved.

Now that you see how the Medicare program is set up, the question that you might want to ask is: How well is it working? The answer depends on what you want it to accomplish. Obviously, Medicare cannot keep people from dying, nor can it keep people from aging and developing chronic illnesses.

Any controversy about how well Medicare is working revolves around how much it costs now and how much it is projected to cost in future years. It is the health policy makers who are engaged in this debate. Most Medicare enrollees like it just the way it is.

According to Medicare Trustee calculations, in 2014 the Medicare program enrolled 54 million persons at the cost of $583 billion; by 2030 the program is projected to enroll double the number of people who were enrolled in 2000. In other words, enrollment is increasing at a rapid rate from year to year. Spending on average is substantially higher for the oldest enrollees. In 2006, the expenditure for beneficiaries ages sixty-five to seventy-four amounted to $5,887 per year; for those over eighty-five, it was $12,059 per year. There is clear evidence showing that only a small proportion of enrollees account for the majority of expenditures. In 2006, spending for those in the top 10 percent of the Medicare expenditures averaged $48,210, in contrast to those in the bottom 90 percent for whom the average cost of coverage was $3,910.

The fact that the baby boom generation has entered its golden years as of 2011 explains why expenditure projections have been attracting the attention of policy experts and politicians who must sign off on funding. Consider these two facts: a) about 76 million people were born between 1946 and 1964; b) the fastest growing age group in the population is the over eighty-five group.

After hearing why policy makers are so concerned about costs, we should stop to note an important positive observation about the way the program operates—it carries out its administrative responsibilities at a cost of 2 percent of program expenditures. On the not-so-positive side, Medicare fraud is growing into a vast industry that is very difficult to control. Now that the outlines of the Medicare program are clear—both its strengths and its weaknesses—the question is, what impact will health care reform have on the Medicare program?

MEDICARE AND HEALTH CARE REFORM

The reform law introduced a large number of changes in the Medicare program, some quite broad and some very specific. Medicare serves as a powerful instrument for shaping health care arrangements in this country for a number of reasons. Medicare rules are the same throughout the country, it enrolls so many people, and it provides such a large share of the payments providers depend on. As you will recall, Medicare came up with the hospital and medical reimbursement formulas, DRGs and RBRVS, which private insurance incorporated as well. Accordingly, Medicare decisions have national policy implications. It is worth noting, however, that the agency does not initiate major changes. Congress does that. Medicare simply carries out the regulations.

Returning to the four basic parts of the program, the changes the ACA introduced include the following:

Part A: There is no premium for Part A. (Remember this is considered an *entitlement*.) Enrollees pay nothing for Part A unless they are admitted to a hospital or other facility. In that case, there is a deductible, which may change from year to year. As of 2015, it was set at $1,260.

Part B: The premium is $104.90 as of 2015 for everyone who earns $85,000 or under. (The 2010 premium was $110.50. It was lowered as a result of greater efficiencies.) The premium goes up as income goes up in five tiers. Those at the highest income level, with earnings over $214,000 on an individual basis, have a monthly deduction of $335.70. In addition to the monthly premium, enrollees pay an annual deductible of $147 and coinsurance, which is generally 20 percent of all Medicare-approved doctor and outpatient charges.

Part C: The changes to Medicare Advantage are extensive:

- The biggest change is the reduction in the overpayment Medicare Advantage plans have been receiving. The law specified that the plans are to receive a maximum overpayment of 2 percent.
- Plans must maintain an 85 percent medical-loss ratio, leaving 15 percent for profit and administration. If a plan exceeds this ratio for two years, Medicare will terminate the contract.
- Payment for services is set using average Medicare costs by county. Plans operating in the most costly counties are to receive 95 percent of the county benchmark; those in lowest-cost counties are to receive 115 percent.
- Plans are to be rated for quality using a five-star rating system established the year before the law was passed. Plans receiving a

rating of four or more stars were scheduled to receive bonus payments starting in 2012, which increase over following years.

- Higher payments based on a risk score formula are to be paid to cover the costs of treating for patients with chronic illnesses.

Part D: Significant changes are being made to the drug benefit section of Medicare:

- All enrollees whose drug costs fell into the doughnut hole received a $250 rebate in the fall of 2010.
- Enrollees whose drug costs fell into the doughnut hole as of 2011 received a 50 percent discount on brand-name drugs and a reduction in coinsurance on generic drugs.
- The doughnut hole is being gradually reduced, meaning that by 2020 enrollees will pay 25 percent coinsurance for drugs rather than 100 percent once their expenditures hit the doughnut hole.
- Subsidies for low-income beneficiaries are being introduced and some payment arrangements that apply to the Indian Health Service are being altered.

The law also introduces changes in how doctors are paid. For example, reimbursement to primary care physicians is being increased; and, annual wellness and prevention visits are covered, meaning that physicians are now being paid for those visits. Physicians practicing in health professional shortage areas are being paid 10 percent more than those in non-shortage areas. A pilot program was initiated aimed at "bundling" services for an episode of care starting at the acute stage when the patient enters the hospital through the outpatient stage. This is designed to produce cost savings by delivering care in a more coordinated way. Let's return to this innovation in chapter 9.

Some of the other broad changes include the creation of a new Independent Payment Advisory Board (IPAB) charged with finding ways to reduce Medicare spending if spending exceeds the targeted growth rate. As of 2017, the spending rate was supposed to be fixed at the annual rate of increase in the Consumer Price Index (CPI) plus one point. However, according to David Blumenthal and David Squires, writing in the Commonwealth Fund blog on January 8, 2015, no committee members had been appointed yet. While some observers expect to see that happen in the not too distant future, ACA opponents have ramped up efforts to have this part of the law dropped.

A number of new rules have been introduced aimed at preventing fraud, such as requiring providers to have face-to-face encounters with patients before certifying the need for home health services and requiring providers to be prepared to provide documentation upon request.

MEDICAID

The other major public program, legislated at the same time as Medicare as an amendment (Title 19) to the Social Security Act, was Medicaid. Its first full year of operation was also 1967. Medicaid is a joint federal-state program created to provide health care services for particular categories of low-income people. They were initially classified into three groups: the poor elderly, people with disabilities too disabled to work, and poor single parents, generally women, with small children. Able-bodied adults, male and female, with no small children, no matter how poor, were ineligible.

The federal government allowed states a fair amount of leeway in determining eligibility based on income. States were permitted to set the eligibility cutoff at a percent of the poverty level established by the federal government for the year, well above or well below that figure (as low as 24% of poverty in some states). The federal government was picking up half of each state's Medicaid outlay, more if the state had an especially high proportion of poor people. This averages out to 57 percent of Medicaid costs across the states. Congress periodically enacted new requirements linked to expanded federal support. By 2003 the federal government had legislated a series of changes to the original law requiring states to provide coverage for twenty-eight additional specific categories of people and allowed states to choose to cover up to twenty-one optional eligibility groups.[5] For example, the federal government began requiring coverage for children under age six and pregnant women who were at 133 percent of poverty or under. Coverage for children under age eighteen who were at 100 percent of poverty was also mandated. States were permitted to cover both parents and children in low-income families if they chose to do so.

The Medicaid program has experienced tremendous expansion and is now the largest of the three public programs, with an enrollment of 68 million persons as of 2011. It costs $415 billion to operate. (Remember the Medicare program enrolls 51 million persons and costs $583 billion.)

While all beneficiaries are entitled to use health care services, they do not necessarily all seek health care. So it is important to look at who is receiving Medicaid services. The statistics for 2008 are as follows:

- The largest percentage out of four eligible categories of Medicaid *enrollees* were children (47.8%) and adults eligible for the Temporary Assistance to Needy Families (TANF; 22%) versus the other two categories, that is, blind and disabled (14.8%) and aged (7.1%).
- This is in contrast to *recipients* of services—the disabled (43.7%) and aged (20.7%) versus children (19.3%) and adults receiving TANF (12.7%).

This is not to criticize how the funds are distributed. It is to correct the widespread assumption that poor women and children are primarily responsible for Medicaid expenditures. Also worth noting is the fact that the top five percent of Medicaid enrollees account for 50 percent of expenditures. Why the funds are allocated in this way is not hard to understand, once you start thinking about it. The disabled and elderly, who are chronically ill, are much more likely to require expensive care. Some people qualify for both Medicare and Medicaid. They are called "dual eligibles." However, the number of elderly who are poor enough to be covered by Medicaid has been declining. So why does Medicaid spend so much on their care? A major part of the answer is that the money is largely spent on nursing home care.

Remember that Medicare covers nursing home care for a limited period of time and only after hospitalization. What about people who need nursing care because they are chronically ill, frail, confused, and need help medicating themselves, toileting, eating, and so forth? The determination that the person needs long-term nursing home care in such cases is made by the family, and a period of hospitalization may not be involved. How is nursing home care paid for under these circumstances? People who are incapacitated enough to go into a nursing home give up whatever money they have to their children, which makes them impoverished and eligible for Medicaid. The only other option is to pay for it out of one's own pocket. Considering that, according to HHS, nursing home care averaged about $6,965 per month for a private room with no added services in 2010, while Medicaid coverage is free, you can understand why Medicaid has become a major alternative and is now providing coverage for an increasing number of people in nursing homes.[6] The disabled category has been growing as well because increasing numbers of people are meeting the criteria for disability.

Persons who fit into one of the approved Medicaid categories must prove that they are poor. Obviously, this means that they must have incomes below whatever the state has set up as the cutoff. That is considerably more complicated than it might first appear. What if a person receives a pension the person can live on, but runs up such high medical bills that he or she ends up being impoverished with very little money left to live on? This is called the "spend down" provision. A person may become eligible because so much of his or her money (e.g., social security check and/or pension) is going to pay for medical bills.

Consider the full implications of Medicaid eligibility. A person must cash in everything she owns before she can say she is truly impoverished. ("She" is appropriate here because there are more poor elderly women than men; because they outlive men and they earn less, they have less of a savings cushion.) That, of course, means that the person can't own a house, a car that is worth more than whatever the state decides, and so on. Finally, the person must prove that he or she is poor. That is the "means testing" feature of the program. Means testing is used to determine whether a person is as poor as he or she claims to be. Accordingly, all financial records must be submitted to the state agency that carries out the review. The standard cutoff has long been $5,000 but is now $6,000 in some states, meaning that one must "cash in," typically giving to one's children everything that might put one's "wealth" over that line.

Critics of the Medicaid program have argued that means testing is a particularly objectionable feature of the program. They say that it is degrading and stigmatizing to have to prove that one is poor. Accordingly, many states no longer require additional proof that one has no wealth and even allow people to keep a car, if the income level is sufficiently low. Others object to the cost of checking to determine if people are eligible for government-covered health care services. Medicaid administrative costs are difficult to assess. However, it is not hard to see why administrative costs would be significant considering how much paperwork and clerical time is involved in attempting to verify eligibility. Administrators of clinics that provide health care to the poor say that about a third of the premiums such organizations receive from government programs are wasted because they are used to cover the administrative costs of re-enrolling people.[7] Critics call this practice "churning."

MEDICAID AND HEALTH CARE REFORM

Medicaid was scheduled to be expanded to all persons under age sixty-five with incomes under 133 percent of poverty as of 2014. The way this is calculated increases this figure to 138 percent of poverty. Adults with no dependent children and women who are not pregnant with incomes below this poverty level were to be covered for the first time in many states. Men without dependent children, obviously most men, were not eligible for Medicaid under the law unless states allowed it

Some governors made it clear that they were opposed to the mandates imposed by the ACA and would not extend Medicaid in their states. In fact, days after the law was passed, 26 states filed or participated in filing lawsuits challenging implementation of the ACA. The Supreme Court handed down its ruling in June 2012 upholding the constitutionality of the both individual mandate and employer mandate, but ruling the Medicaid expansion unconstitutional. The governors of states involved in the suit objected to the requirement that they create Health Exchanges in order to keep the Medicaid funding they were already receiving. The Supreme Court decision meant that states would not have to expand their Medicaid programs and enroll more people. The decision meant that states would not have to set up Health Exchanges and the Medicaid funds they were already getting would not be withdrawn as the penalty for not setting up an exchange. (As you will recall from chapter 1, the Obama administration did not expect this ruling and was not ready to create federal Health Exchanges in twenty-six states. The disastrous rollout was the result.)

Governors in other states were not so much opposed to the law but feared that they would not have the funds to implement the Medicaid reform due to financial difficulties brought on by the recession.

In order to reduce resistance to compliance, the federal government made funds available to states to cover 100 percent of the cost of health care services for all new enrollees from 2014 through 2016, 95 percent in 2017, gradually dropping that rate over the following years to 90 percent by 2020. The health care reform legislation made clear that undocumented illegal immigrants were not being covered by the expanded Medicaid law.

In order to ensure that physicians would be willing to accept the new influx of Medicaid enrollees the ACA raised primary care physician payments to the reimbursement rate set by Medicare.

STATE CHILD HEALTH INSURANCE PROGRAM

The State Child Health Insurance Program (CHIP, originally SCHIP) or Title 21 of the Social Security Act is the third major public health program. It was passed in conjunction with the budget reform legislation of 1997. It was legislated in response to what everyone who looks at health insurance and poverty data realized some time ago: that poor and near-poor children are at particularly high risk of being uninsured. CHIP provides federal funds to insure children under the age of nineteen whose family income is under 200 percent of the federal poverty level, which is much higher than the Medicaid cutoff in the majority of states. There is general support for providing health insurance for children; however, the challenge of enrolling children in families in which the adults are not poor enough to qualify for Medicaid has not been easy. States use three different models for establishing and administering CHIP: 1) a separate CHIP program, 2) Medicaid expansion, and 3) some combination of these. As of 2013, the percentage of eligible children who are enrolled stands at 88.3 percent; however, 4 million eligible children are still uninsured.[8] The law was scheduled to expire in September 2015 but was reauthorized in April 2015 for the next two years.

At the time the CHIP legislation was passed, Congress appropriated $40 billion over ten years that states could use to provide health care services for enrolled children with the provision that the states had to have administrative procedures in place and were already enrolling children. It took some states longer to do this than anticipated, which meant that allocated funds were not spent. That led to new controversies. A number of states that created CHIP programs more quickly applied for the unspent funds to cover childless adults. Some policy makers objected, saying that this was a distortion of the intent of the law. Congress dealt with the problem of unspent funds by passing a so-called SCHIP Fix in 2003, which allowed states to access some of the remaining unspent funds. It appears that a great deal of attention was directed at analyzing the structure of the programs by state and distribution of these funds rather than measuring impact. That can be explained in part by the fact that there is general agreement that CHIP is beneficial where it is operating effectively. The primary concern has been getting it to operate effectively, that is, enroll all eligible children.

REMAINING DISCUSSION POINTS

The primary question that policy makers confront is how to cut the cost of public health insurance programs. Because the three programs have been institutionalized, and even treated as entitlements by some, it makes arguing to abolish them politically risky to politicians determined to cut government expenditures. However, the concern about public debt in Washington, DC, if not the rest of the country, in the spring of 2011, finally allowed for the initiation of discussion on cutting back on the costs of these programs. Let's consider some of the proposed solutions.

One of the options explored was raising the age of eligibility to qualify for Medicare from sixty-five to sixty-seven in 2014. That had already been done in the case of Social Security, so why not do it in the case of Medicare? The following is based on a Kaiser Family Foundation Program on Medicare Policy report issued in 2011.[9]

Here are the facts. You can decide whether it would be a good move. Raising the age of eligibility by two years would generate an estimated $7.6 billion in net Medicare savings to the federal government. It would require a drop in coverage for about 5 million persons in this age bracket. However, it is projected that the savings would be offset by the $8.9

billion the government would have to spend for those who would then have to be covered by Medicaid; plus the $7.5 billion that the federal government would be providing in tax credits to those buying insurance through exchanges; and by the $7 billion reduction in Medicare premium receipts. The burden would shift $4.5 billion to employers who would still be the primary providers of insurance for their workers. Everyone buying insurance through exchanges, that would now include sixty-five- and sixty-six-year-olds, would pay 3 percent more for coverage because of increased risk of illness in the risk pool; Part B enrollees would also pay 3 percent more because younger Medicare recipients would be out of the risk pool; and states would have to spend $7 billion to provide Medicaid coverage for the new enrollees.

In short, Medicare expenditures would certainly drop. However, costs would not be eliminated; they would be shifted. What does this cautionary tale tell us? Cost shifting does not achieve cost savings and may even increase government spending.

QUESTIONS AND ISSUES TO THINK ABOUT

- There has been little controversy about funding the CHIP program, which provides health insurance for children whose parents' earnings are under 200 percent of poverty. Most people, including politicians, support the program. But, it does not cover all eligible children. What do you think explains why so many children are not enrolled in the program? What alternatives would you suggest to fix this?
- Medicare Advantage was created based on the idea that the private sector would attain greater efficiencies than traditional Medicare. Consider how efficient Medicare is and how efficient Medicare Advantage is. What indicator would you use to determine efficiency?
- Medicare was specifically prohibited from entering into negotiations with pharmaceutical companies over the price of pharmaceuticals. What do you think are the pros and cons of this proscription?

7

THE HEALTH CARE SYSTEMS IN OTHER COUNTRIES

As you will recall, the health care system satisfaction survey discussed in chapter 1 indicated that people in the other countries being surveyed do not think their health care systems are perfect, but they are much less dissatisfied than people in the United States. You might wonder what it is that that people in other countries like about their health care arrangements. Looking at it from a sociological perspective, the satisfaction that other countries are registering may be because they have been better at incorporating their distinctive building blocks, that is, social values and expectations, in constructing their health care systems. We see this very clearly in the following narratives describing how the systems evolved. The accounts reveal a couple of other things, for one, other countries developed their health care arrangements in an unsystematic manner, just like we did; and, they continue to introduce health care system reforms on a regular but unsystematic basis, again like we are doing. Other countries are simply doing a better job in meeting their citizens' values and expectations than the United States is doing. Moreover, they are achieving better outcomes at lower cost. How that can happen is worth examining more closely, isn't it?

THE UNITED STATES COMPARED TO OTHER COUNTRIES

When policy makers in this country discuss the changes that we need to make to improve our health care system, they typically refer to a small number of countries, those mentioned in the first chapter, to make comparisons. Various observers and commentators have been eager to point out what is wrong with health care arrangements in virtually every other country and to argue that we would be making a big mistake if we imported any of their arrangements, except maybe for the Swiss system. Back to that in a moment.

Whenever talk about reform moves to center stage, the health care arrangements in two countries, Canada and the UK, get most attention. The worst charge that critics can launch is to say that their health care systems are socialistic. As we know this is meant to invoke images of failure, grinding bureaucracy, and incompetence.

Since it is the Canadian system that consistently inspires especially heated debate in this country, let's look at their arrangements first. (The figures on per person expenditures for all the countries discussed below come from the World Bank, averaged for 2009–2013. The life expectancy figures are from the CIA for 2014. Unless otherwise indicated, general information is based on the Commonwealth Fund, 2013 survey.)

Canada

As of 2014, Canadian men were living to 79.07 and women to 84.42 and paying $5,741 per person. By comparison, the United States was spending $8,895 per person; men were living to 77.11 and women to 81.94 during this period. You have to admit, they must be doing something right.

Canada has ten provinces, which are like our states but more independent of the federal government than American states, and three territories (the Yukon Territory, the Northwest Territories, and Nunavut). The foundation for the present health care system was laid in 1867 when the federal government gave the provinces responsibility for health care. However, the Canadian system really took shape during the 1940s. The province of Saskatchewan was the first to enact a provincial hospital insurance plan in 1947. In 1957, the federal government passed legislation establishing a national program. By 1961 all the provinces had signed on. That same year the federal government agreed to pay half the costs. The financial windfall of federal support for hospital insurance caused Saskatchewan to propose a new program to cover medical care costs (i.e., doctors' fees). The doctors were not happy about the hospital plan; however, they were far less happy about the medical portion of the plan. They said that this was the beginning of socialized medicine, which would cause quality to decline, costs to go up because of mismanagement, and treatments to be determined by bureaucrats. The citizens of the province thought otherwise. Saskatchewan introduced medical insurance in 1961. The other provinces followed. And by 1971, Canada had a National Health Insurance Program called Medicare.

Let's stop for a moment to consider why Saskatchewan was the first to embrace hospital insurance. There is a particularly interesting set of social values that provide the building block for establishing a provincial hospital plan that is worth examining more closely. Saskatchewan is a wheat-growing province. For all you city dwellers, what do you think the growers do with the wheat they harvest? They don't take it to the local grocery store or farmers' market to sell. It has to be processed. And they don't install a wheat-processing plant in their backyards. Even if they could process it themselves, how would they organize packaging it and selling it, getting bids on it outside of their own community, delivering it, and so on? The answer is that growers in each community got together years ago and created cooperative processing plants that sell the wheat to wholesalers who buy from many co-ops and sell it in bulk to companies that make bakery products, cereals, and so on. Now here is the important point. Each grower is paid based on the weight of the wheat he brings. The manager of the co-op does the weighing and pays according to the weight. All the growers are closely involved in the operations of the co-op because their livelihood depends on how well it functions. They determine who will serve as co-op manager; they decide whether any of the equipment needs to replaced or repaired, and so on.

Does that help explain why a hospital insurance plan to which everyone would contribute and which would cover everyone in the province developed here? Extending this account, what does the fact that the other provinces were quick to adopt both hospital insurance and medical insurance tell you about the Canadian value system? Yes, there was some opposition, but you have to admit that they succeeded in working that out and got the legislation passed at rocket speed compared to how long it is taking the United States to provide insurance for everyone in the country.

The Canadian Medicare plan has a number of distinguishing features. It is generally referred to as a "single-payer" plan. The single payer is, of course, the government. Coverage must be comprehensive as specified by federal law, but additional services, such as dental benefits, home care, and drugs, are offered at the discretion of the province. Insurance offered by private insurance companies is legal in provinces that do not provide for such services. The vast majority of hospitals are privately owned and operated by nonprofit organizations. Most doctors are paid on a fee-for-service basis, although an increasing number are opting to be paid on a salary basis. Patients are free to choose any primary care doctor they want. Canadians are issued a Medicare card, which is like a credit card. Patients are not billed, because doctors' and hospital charges are reimbursed directly by the government.

We have a lot in common with Canadians. We share a very lengthy border. We speak the same language. We have similar historical roots. People in other countries can't tell us apart from the Canadians. So if we are so much like them and their health care arrangements are superior to ours in many ways—they spend less than we do, everyone is fully covered, they live a little longer than we do, and they seem to be quite satisfied—why don't we just copy it and be done with it? The answer is that no matter how alike we seem to be on the outside, the Canadian plan reflects their values, which are not our values. Even if some people in this country would like for the United States to embrace their values, that is not the way it works. Consider some of the objections heard in this country.

In the Canadian system everyone is covered by the same plan, which means you cannot buy more, faster, or better care. Americans refuse to accept that kind of arrangement. The majority of Canadians take the position that, "when everyone is in the same boat, that boat is likely to be much better cared for." In other words, it is always easier to deny funding to "them," but when it is "us" whose care is at stake, "we" tend to exhibit more concern and readiness to treat the topic of the need for increased funding more seriously.

Canadians debate what they call "privatization" of services, that is, for-profit health care services governed by market forces. The same arguments prevail in Canada as here, namely, that for-profit sector organizations are superior, less expensive, and more attentive to consumer preferences. Opponents argue that anything that is not accessible to the entire population violates the spirit of the law that created the Canadian Medicare system.

The growing number of free-standing for-profit CT and MRI clinics that provide imaging services, which people must pay for out of their own pockets, indicates that privatization is moving ahead. Access to faster service for a fee has received greater attention in recent years because of growing dissatisfaction with the length of waiting times for tests, including CT and MRI scans.

The length of waiting time for CT and MRI scans is related to a significant feature of the Canadian system, namely the "cap" on funding. Each year the provincial government sets a health care budget. Hospitals receive a fixed amount of money that covers basic operating expenses plus inflation, but they must negotiate any major expenses separately. The state of the province's finances and the positon taken by its political leadership determine how generous the province is in agreeing to fund additional hospital expenditures for technology and other kinds of upgrades.

Doctors do not have to negotiate over fees from year to year. Their fees are reimbursed in full for all the charges they submit. Why doesn't this result in unlimited charges? One reason is that doctors, particularly specialists, have increasingly been opting to be reimbursed on a non-fee-for-service basis. They sign a fixed annual contract with the hospital where they do most of their work. Those who rely on fee-for-service reimbursement accept lower levels of reimbursement after reaching specified income levels in some but not all provinces. For example, in 2004, doctors in Ontario, which is the richest province, agreed to accept 75 percent of the scheduled fee after reaching $465,000. Doctors' fee schedules are determined through negotiation between each respective provincial government and provincial medical society. The provincial government does not run out of funds for the year because it has budgeted what it will be spending based on the record of expenditures over the previous year and the revenue it expects to collect.

As an aside, some states in this country do run out of funds. They deal with this by putting off paying their bills. Delaying Medicaid payments to doctors and hospitals until the following year is a common tactic. If their finances do not improve, they repeat the same pattern the following year, possibly over multiple years.

Canadian patients do not refer themselves to specialists. They see family practitioners for routine care who refer patients to specialists when they determine that it is necessary. Specialists are not eager to see patients who self-refer. The explanation is that specialists are paid a higher fee for referred patients, but are paid the same fee as family practitioners for patients who are not referred. This arrangement gets further reinforcement from the fact that family practitioners stop referring to specialists who do not observe this norm.

American doctors have traditionally considered Canadian reimbursement arrangements to be an unacceptable intrusion on the part of the government. Canadian doctors see it as preferable to the constant "micromanagement" that American doctors have to endure from insurance companies. They say that American doctors have to get preapproval from patients' insurance companies to make sure the insurance plan covers the procedure so that they will be paid for performing the procedure. Because there are so many plans with so many variations in coverage that may change at any time, doctors cannot easily avoid this step. One or two medical associations and organizations in this country periodically issue statements indicating support for the Canadian single-payer approach.

Canadian doctors are willing to accept a cap on income or a set salary because of two notable differences in expenses faced by Canadian doctors in contrast to American doctors. American doctors typically enter into practice with a large educational debt. Canadian medical schools are heavily subsidized by the government, meaning that medical school tuition runs anywhere from $5,000 to $15,000 or so per year, depending on the province. As you know, this is in sharp contrast to how much American medical education costs. Also, malpractice insurance is much lower in Canada. In large part, this is because contingency fees are considered unethical or illegal in Canada. (Remember the contingency fee that goes to lawyers in this country is generally a third or a quarter of the settlement, depending on whether the case is settled in or out of court and no fee if they lose the case.)

Canadians find themselves periodically arguing about the performance of their health care system because the provinces have, from time to time, had to decide whether they wanted to come up with additional funding or cut services. The federal contribution to health care costs, which was 50 percent originally, was cut during the 1980s, finally dropping to 25 percent by the early 1990s. As you might imagine, talking about how to compensate for lost funds opened up public debate as to where the money would come from. This led to highly charged questions about what should be cut to lower costs and whether to allow more health care services to be offered for an additional charge. The fact that Canada was faced with an economic recession during the early 1990s led to the fear that the health care system was threatened. The economy improved during the last years of the twentieth century. In 1999, the federal government announced a fiscal surplus, which everyone agreed should go to the provinces to cover Medicare.[1]

As concern about funding declined during the first decade of the twenty-first century so has the volume of debate about how to best save the health care system. Polls have long found Canadians expressing strong support for maintaining the status quo on the essence of the single-payer arrangement, meaning they overwhelmingly reject two-tier care and user fees for core services.

To sum up, the most important differences between the Canadian system and ours is that theirs is a single-payer, capped system, while ours depends on market forces and competition to control costs; theirs provides health care coverage for everyone, ours does not; and theirs costs less than ours. These points speak to costs and access, but what about quality? Their life expectancy and infant mortality rates are better than ours. This, of course, just scratches the surface of things that people can argue about in discussing the differences between their system and our system.

Let's turn to England to see how their health care system compares to ours.

England

As of 2014, men in England were living to 78.07, women to 82.69, and paying $3,647 per person. (The U.S. rates are 77.11, 81.94, and $8,895.)

England, Scotland, Wales, and Northern Ireland together make up the United Kingdom. Because the health care systems are not identical throughout the UK, the following discussion focuses on England, where health insurance for workers came into existence about 1911. Health care for the rest of the family was not the employer's responsibility. The logic is clear. Remember, England was the place the industrial revolution began. The industrialists were interested in making sure that their workers were healthy. Their main concern was workforce stability, not anyone's health per se, and certainly not the health of persons who were not their employees.

The emergence of hospitals in England has a longer history. This history serves as a particularly graphic illustration of how social values influence the development of social institutions.[2] Hospitals were established several centuries ago (some as early as the sixteenth and seventeenth centuries) with the express purpose of serving three separate segments of the population. The aristocracy went to sanatoriums, which were located in the countryside where the patients could benefit from clean air and the special comforts the rich expected. The working poor (i.e., all workers, in contrast to the aristocracy who do not work even now) went to voluntary hospitals often operated by religious orders. That left the "undeserving poor" (i.e., those who were too sick, too old, or too disabled to work). Because the aristocracy would not mix with the working poor and neither would mix with the undeserving poor, each segment had to have its own hospital. All that changed with World War II.

During the war, the government mapped out all the hospitals and counted all the hospital beds in the country and mandated that 10 percent of the beds in each hospital be set aside for military use, abolishing the differences across the three types of hospitals. The hospitals were paid a per diem (daily) rate whether the bed was in use or not. Everyone in the country was making sacrifices. This was the hospitals' contribution to the war effort. While the country came out of the war victorious, it sustained heavy damage and was broke. The government proposed taking over responsibility for the entire health care system as a reward to the public for making enormous sacrifices during the wartime period. In other words, from that time on, the government took over ownership of the whole health care system. Not everyone was entirely happy about this plan. Doctors were especially loud in their objections. They said the government's plan was socialized medicine and would bring with it the downfall of professional medical practice. Looking at it objectively, it was, for better or worse, a major step toward socialized medicine. Doctors objected to being salaried instead of being paid as professionals under the traditional fee-for-service arrangement. Still, one has to be practical in these matters. Having the government provide a guaranteed income was not easy to dismiss given the postwar state of affairs.

The solution was interesting. The general practitioners agreed to be paid under a *capitation* arrangement. They acceded to having X number of patients (around 2,000 depending on whether the practice was in an urban or rural area) sign up with them for care and get paid "by the head" (i.e., capitation) whether those patients came to see them or not. This meant that the doctors were guaranteed a steady income. The patients were guaranteed the services of a doctor. Patients had the opportunity to change doctors once a year by signing up with a new doctor of their choice. The specialists made a different bargain. They agreed to be salaried and work for a particular hospital in return for having access to 10 percent of the beds in that hospital for their private patients, whom they could bill separately. Everyone else working in the hospital had always been salaried, so that did not change.

In short, England has had a National Health Service, the NHS (not a national health insurance system), since 1948, with everyone in the country having full access to health care services. In assuming responsibility for the hospitals as of 1948, the government took over ownership of all the hospitals and clinics. It pays everyone who works for the NHS. And, as you recall from the first chapter, there may be some grumbling about how things work, but only 3 percent of people think the system needs to be totally overhauled. Further evidence of how the Brits feel about the NHS comes from a 2014 survey indicating that it outranks the monarchy in popularity, and the monarchy is very popular for historical and symbolic reasons.[3] And, as some might remember, the Brits exhibited a very public display of affection for the NHS in celebrations during the 2012 Olympics. One regularly hears that the health care system in the UK has all kinds of problems. You certainly don't get that impression when you ask the Brits about it.

A more concrete way of assessing satisfaction is to count how many people opt out of the system. In the case of doctors, how many choose to leave to practice elsewhere? The critics of the NHS say that doctors are leaving in droves. In actuality, it is difficult to know how many leave and for what reasons. There is no count of how many leave and return after some period of postgraduate education or research outside the country (not always to the United States) or a stint in an underserved country. To the extent that evidence exists, very few doctors are leaving.

In the case of patients, the measure is how many choose to buy private insurance and go to private doctors and hospitals. Until the 1980s, only about 5 percent of the population chose to buy private insurance. As of 2012, 11 percent have private insurance.

There is an important feature associated with the purchase of private health insurance that cannot be dismissed. People buy it on top of having access to care through the National Health Service. What advantage are people seeking in buying private insurance if they have access to free care? Better doctors, better technology, more care? Not exactly. The answer is—getting around the "queue," in other words, waiting in line, the same reason Canadians buy private insurance. In order to keep costs down, the NHS prevented people from getting health care services "on demand" (i.e., whenever they feel like it) for problems that are not life threatening. In other words, people must wait while more urgent cases are treated. Those who feel that the wait is too long, and can afford to do so, buy private insurance. One of the most often cited reasons for doing this has been hip replacement surgery. It is painful, but not life threatening.

Now for the essence of the "important feature" I mentioned. Private hospitals, where patients with private insurance go, do routine surgeries, like hip replacements. (I know, not routine to the person having the surgery, but routine in terms of how often it is done, and how much risk is involved.) If something does go seriously wrong, the patient is picked up by ambulance and taken to a major NHS hospital, which is equipped to deal with high-risk and complicated problems. So everyone is happy, right? Well, not necessarily.

The reason that people buy private insurance is that the government kept the budget for the NHS low—much too low, in the opinion of some. (England has been spending a little less than half of what we spent for the last two decades of the twentieth century as reflected in percentage of GDP.) Couldn't the British alter this? After all, it is their social institution; they created it, they can change it, right? That is true.

But remember this is the NHS, not a public insurance plan. Its budget is in the hands of the ruling political party in office, which is elected by the public. In theory, the public should be able to convince the government to respond to its demands and allocate more funds for this purpose. The public did demand increased funding during the 1980s, and on one or two occasions the government did respond, but only after an enormous amount of public protest.

A survey conducted during the late 1990s found 69 percent of the British public saying that the government was not improving things enough; physicians reported suffering from low morale.[4] British policy analysts concluded that it is almost as difficult to spend more money effectively in England as it is to control costs in the United States. The basic problem seems to have been that expectations were raised higher than the government could meet.

Because people must weigh their dissatisfaction with the way one social institution is being treated by the government against how they think other social institutions are faring, they may not be so eager to oust the current political party until they are unhappy enough about all of it. They are more apt to try to convince the government via appeals and protests first. When that did not bring the results the public wanted, the British decided that electing a more liberal political party to office would improve the health care system as well as other social arrangements and institutions. They elected a new prime minister in 1997, Tony Blair.

Blair reversed the changes introduced during the two previous Conservative Party administrations, who had been impressed with U.S. efforts to introduce competition in order to increase efficiency. The mechanism the Conservative administrations had developed to promote greater efficiency was "fund holding." This gave general practitioners the option of managing their own funds and spending the monies they saved in running the practice on anything the practice group wanted to purchase. (They could not keep the surplus as a bonus.) Policy makers were somewhat surprised to find that the groups used the funds to ensure that social services were more closely aligned with medical services. The American way would have been to spend it on more technology and more expensive furnishings for their offices to attract more patients—right? It just goes to show how cultural values shape social institutions and how they vary from one country to another.

A number of sweeping changes followed the political shift. New diagnostic and treatment centers were opened to reduce waiting times. A National Institute for Clinical Excellence was established and mandated to issue binding recommendations on the delivery of medical services funded by the NHS. Doctors were now required to go through relicensure every five years. As of April 2004, general practitioners were permitted to choose among a number of contractual incentive arrangements for the first time, including capitation with incentives for reaching particular service targets, for example, a higher vaccination rate. This was part of an effort to reach ten specific targets for quality improvement, such as reducing cancer deaths by 20 percent. Contracts with specialists, called "consultants" in England, have changed only to the extent that NHS patients were now permitted, for the first time, to schedule their own appointments with specialists online.

The election of a Conservative-led coalition government in 2010 brought about a new wave of sweeping changes and has continued to make changes since then. Hospitals were encouraged to separate from the NHS and become independent nonprofit organizations. GPs were given far more authority and funds to negotiate for services to be delivered by hospitals. GPs did not exactly welcome the changes. Many did not believe that they had the administrative background to take on this kind of responsibility and risk. Others said that they expected administrative costs to increase rather than decrease, using the high administrative costs of competition in the United States to make the point. The government has continued to make adjustments. The impact of specific changes is being evaluated.[5]

Germany

As of 2014, German men were living to 78.15, women to 82.86, and paying $4,683 per person.

The German health care system is the oldest national health care system in Europe. It was introduced in 1871 by the government under Otto von Bismarck (in one part of Germany, Prussia), who reasoned that if the government was thought to be meeting the needs of workers as the country went through industrialization, workers would be less likely to support radical political movements, and his government would stay in control. The current system took shape in 1883 with the passage of the Sickness Insurance Act and applied to all of Germany. The law required all workers below a certain income level to join existing mutual benefit societies, which had established branches that dealt with health care, called sickness funds.

Mutual benefit societies created by guilds and, in some cases, villages to cover the costs of such catastrophes as funerals, lost income resulting from a temporary injury, and permanent disability had been in existence for the last two or three hundred years. People set up these funds to meet the needs they thought were most pressing at the time. Coverage for health care was a secondary consideration until much later because the effectiveness of health care was limited and, what there was, was not costly. By the time that the Sickness Insurance Act was passed, 18,942 sickness funds were already in existence, covering 4.7 million people.[6]

The 1883 law gave the funds the authority to establish and operate health clinics. This meant that they were in a position to hire doctors and other staff members. Because the sickness funds were small and run by persons who did not necessarily have the skill to manage large sums of money, doctors were often not paid as promised. They responded by going out on strike whenever that happened. The system could not be described as stable and working to the satisfaction of all involved.[7] Things became more stable during the decade of the 1930s. Interestingly, while doctors were very dissatisfied with prevailing arrangements, they had little influence in shaping the national health insurance system before this time because they had no professional association to represent their views. Germany's doctors organized themselves into a national association in 1931. (Remember, the American Medical Association came into existence in 1847.)

The German health care system evolved as the society modernized, which affected the organization of the sickness funds. The number of sickness funds declined over time as some failed and others merged. As of 2013, the number of funds had dropped to 134.

Clearly, the federal government has been closely involved in shaping the health care system from the beginning. The system is governed by two principles—solidarity and "subsidiarity," which were written into law in 1949 and to which parties across the political spectrum subscribe. The goal was health insurance coverage for everyone in the country. Enrollment did not become mandatory until 2009.

The government sees its role as overseer of the system but does not run the system. It monitors costs and quality. When hospital costs began to rise more rapidly during the mid-1980s, the government stopped paying hospitals whatever they charged and instead required them to operate within a preset budget negotiated at the beginning of the year. This had a significant stabilizing effect. The government adopted the DRG system for calculating hospital costs and uses this to negotiate hospital budgets. Quality of hospital care is evaluated based on information that hospitals are required to submit on twenty-seven indicators. Further evidence of government oversight of quality has to do with drug effectiveness. Pharmaceutical companies are required to submit scientific dossiers on their drugs. The dossiers are evaluated by a federal committee. The government uses this material to negotiate the price of the drugs.

Doctors are either office-based or hospital-based. Their practices do not overlap. The hospital-based doctors are salaried. The salary is set according to the doctor's specialty and years of experience. Office-based doctors are paid on a fee-for-service basis, according to a fee schedule established in negotiations between sickness funds and physicians' groups. The fees are subject to a cap, which works in response to a very interesting and effective mechanism. Medical expenditures are reviewed on a quarterly basis by a unit created by the local medical society. If the total expenditure on office-based physicians' fees exceeds the projected amount, the fees for all office-based practitioners are reduced. Doctors whose fees are significantly higher than those of their colleagues are likely to come under scrutiny—not by bureaucrats, but by a committee of fellow physicians who have the expertise to evaluate the reasons behind the high rate and authority to impose sanctions on doctors found to be "overtreating" patients. That tends to keep the lid on medical expenditures.

It is worth noting that the German system underwent considerable change during the decade of the 1990s. In part, this was a response to the sudden rise in health care costs that resulted from unification and the additional funds that had to be spent to reorganize the system of care found in East Germany to match the highly technologically advanced system in West Germany.

Germany has been interested in how the private market for insurance works in the United States. In addition, it has been willing to experiment as long as competition did not damage the strengths of the existing system and upset major stakeholders. Put that way, one can understand why the German health care system is not changing very radically or very fast.

Japan

U.S. health policy makers do not consider the Japanese system to be a good model. However, since the Japanese have had the longest life expectancy among the most economically advanced countries in the world for the past several decades, exploring how much their health care system has to do with it is something that has attracted the interest of American researchers. As of 2014, men were living to 81.13, and women to 87.99. They were and are spending far less than other advanced countries, at $4,752 per person, to achieve the highest life expectancy in the world.

The Japanese instituted health insurance in 1927. The country achieved universal coverage by 1961. Everyone under the age of 75 is required to enroll in a health insurance plan. There are about 3,500 insurers.

The country is organized into 47 prefectures and 1,700 municipalities. Each prefecture is required to create a cost-control plan. Prefectures may limit use of expensive drugs, delay purchase of expensive equipment, and deny payment for inappropriate services. Municipalities are responsible for insuring everyone over the age of seventy-five and unemployed. Employer-based plans, to which both employees and employers contribute, may be self-funded by employers or government-managed and partially government-subsidized. Plans are closely monitored by the government.

Americans find Japanese health care arrangements very different from ours. But understanding how the Japanese managed to spend so much less per person in 2014 and still achieve the longest life expectancy of any country is worth exploring. One reason they can spend so much less is that they have about one-third less surgery than we do. Part of the explanation for the low surgery rate is that organ replacement is culturally unacceptable and restricted by law.

The fact that Japan built its health care system by grafting Western medical practices onto a system based on oriental, basically Chinese, medicine accounts for the Japanese attitude regarding surgery. Many doctors advocate the use of herbal medications as well as pharmaceuticals used in Western medicine. They not only prescribe, but dispense both kinds of medications. To put this into context, oriental medicine favors medications and discourages surgery. So there is a lot of prescribing.

This does not mean that the Japanese are opposed to diagnostic procedures. They have a larger number of MRI machines than other economically advanced countries. The Japanese have 46.9 machines per million persons; we have 31.5; the Canadians have 8.5; and the UK has 5.9. (Numbers are not available for many other countries.) To the extent that we have information on the number of MRI machines per country, there seems to be no correlation with life expectancy.

It is also true that Japan has been reluctant to lower hospital costs by reducing the length of hospital stays. Japanese patients stay in the hospital far longer than Americans do—during the mid-1990s the U.S. average length of stay was 5.1 days while theirs ranged from 15.8 to 29.1 days depending on the hospital. This is explained, in part, by the fact that the Japanese have not been ready to build nursing homes for extended-stay patients. Remember, this is a far more traditional society than ours, where women have historically stayed home and cared for aging parents and sick relatives. More women are now working, but the health care delivery system has not caught up. People dealt with the change in women's roles by checking in their elderly relatives for an extended stay when the work of caring for the aging relative has gotten too burdensome or when they went on vacation.

In the spring of 2000, the government agreed to do something about the problem. It passed legislation funding long-term care for the elderly. However, there are very few nursing homes ready to accept elderly patients and Japanese society is not entirely prepared to institutionalize elderly relatives. The shift in attitude and behavior is expected to move forward slowly, making the transition manageable both socially and financially.

Are there lessons to be learned from the Japanese? By the way, I won't let you dismiss the differences by saying that it is their diet. Yes, their diet plays a critical role; that cannot be denied. But their diet has not changed very much over the last three or four decades when their life expectancy skyrocketed to the top of the international life expectancy scales. It is also true that they have long led the world in the rate of stomach cancer; they smoke at an incredibly high rate, at least the men do; their cities have been highly polluted in the past and are still very crowded; and they work long hours and take little time off, to name a few things that you might expect to detract from their good health. I leave you to ponder these inconsistencies. If you decide to explore this issue in greater detail I recommend that you consider the answer offered by an increasing number of researchers; they believe that social arrangements across social institutions have more to do with the health status of a country's inhabitants than its health care system, which, as a single social institution, cannot overcome factors linked to ill health associated with the operations of other social institutions in the country.[8]

How does this manifest itself? Health policy analysts say that the Japanese spend less on health care services because they don't have our social problems. They have very little poverty and far less violence, which requires expensive health services, especially emergency room care.

Switzerland

Let's consider why some health policy experts were campaigning to have the United States adopt the Swiss system during the debates on health care system reform prior to passage of the ACA. As of 2014, men were living to 80.1 and the women to 84.81, giving them the second longest life expectancy after Japan. In terms of GDP, in 2011, they were spending 11 percent while we were spending 17.7 percent. Their life expectancy rate and GDP were offered as reasons to adopt the Swiss system. The Swiss system was then and is now the third most expensive among economically advanced countries, at $8,890 per person; Norway's is next at $5,669. Ours is, of course, the most expensive at $8,895. However, the primary reason policy makers were arguing for the Swiss system was that people are free to choose the plan they want. Insurance is purchased on an individual basis from private sector companies.

A closer look at how the Swiss plan evolved and how it operates reveals that the freedom to choose one's own health insurance plan is more constrained than it first appears.[9] The system went through a major reform in 1996, when purchase of health insurance became compulsory for everyone in the country, including every child. What spurred the reform was objection to the fact that women were being charged more for insurance coverage. The reform meant that everyone pays the same premium for a basic plan. The price of the policy may vary based on the how high the deductible is for the plan. A government committee determines what services are covered. The committee relies heavily on evidence-based research, often conducted in other countries.

The system is closely monitored. The enforcement of the individual mandate makes that clear. Every individual must register with the canton in which he or she resides. There are twenty-six cantons responsible for licensing providers, hospital planning, and subsidizing those who need help paying for insurance. If an individual does not purchase insurance coverage, the canton selects a plan for the person and bills the person.

The main reason health reform architects in the United States were forced to reject the Swiss plan has to do with out-of-pocket costs. The Swiss system includes a variety of copayments, for routine medical care, drugs, hospital stays. That means that the Swiss pay for about 20 percent of their health care out-of-pocket. Americans pay about 11.6 percent and are registering considerable dissatisfaction about how much they are paying. The Swiss system was a nonstarter once the majority of American policy makers became aware of that. As you will recall, only 8 percent of the Swiss are registering dissatisfaction with this arrangement and want to see the system totally dismantled. Social scientists say that we must recognize the fact that there is very little poverty in Switzerland and that this explains why so many Swiss people are not displeased about the cost of their health care arrangements.

The fact that some politicians in this country were arguing for a Swiss system has inspired policy researchers to continue weighing the advantages and disadvantages of its health system. A recent analysis of the Swiss and Dutch systems, both of which rely on "managed competition," indicates that their health care expenditures are considerably higher than the average for other economically advanced countries.[10] In comparing hospital administrative costs across eight countries, the researchers who conducted that study found "managed competition" arrangements that rely on competition to correlate with much higher administrative costs. In fact, they say, the greater the reliance on competition, the higher the comparative costs. They interpret their results to mean that "the reduction of administrative costs would best be accomplished through the use of a simpler and less market-oriented payment scheme."[11]

France

As of 2014, men were living to 78.55 and women to 84.91, and paying $4,690 per person.

Although U.S. policy makers are not interested in debating the strengths and weaknesses of the French system, policy makers regularly mention what it is about the system that is causing the World Health Organization to nominate it as the best health care system in the world. Briefly: basic health insurance coverage is mandatory and linked to occupation. It is obtained through a person's employer. Both the employer and employee share the cost. Individuals may purchase supplementary insurance on top of the basic plan through employment as well. This allows the person to cover additional costs or copayments for office visits, drugs, hospitalization, and so on. Their out-of-pocket costs run about 7 percent. Exemptions for a variety of reasons, for instance, low income, specific diseases, and certain hospital treatments mean that there is no cost sharing given those circumstances.

As of 2000, those whose income falls under a certain cutoff have been entitled to free insurance coverage. Others have been eligible for financial assistance since 2005 to enable them to purchase insurance. The result is—everyone in the country is covered by health insurance. That does not make France unique, since virtually all highly industrialized countries insure everyone in the country.

The explanation for the WHO's rationale for nominating France as the country with the best health care system is that it achieves the lowest number of *preventable* deaths in comparison to other highly advanced countries. This is known as the "amenable mortality" measure. As of 2003, France had 67 avoidable deaths per 100,000 while the United States had 110 such deaths per 100,000.[12] Given the satisfaction survey results we saw in the first chapter, that only 11 percent say that the system requires total reorganization, we can conclude that they are quite satisfied with these arrangements.

WHAT ARE WE TO CONCLUDE ABOUT OTHER COUNTRIES' SYSTEMS?

Now that we have discussed the systems in the countries that policy analysts mention most often in comparison to the United States' system, are you ready to take a quiz? You might enjoy testing your knowledge by taking the quiz offered by the Commonwealth Fund in conjunction with a report entitled: "Health Care Around the World: How Much Do You Know?"[13]

Returning to our discussion, we can see that the countries we looked at started dealing with concerns about health care at a different time in history and for somewhat different reasons. Once the foundations of their systems were in place, they just built on top of those foundations. Retrospectively, we can see that the decade of the 1960s, the mid-1980s, and, most recently, during the years just before and after the turn of the twenty-first century, brought forth notable reforms in a number of countries.

The 1960s signaled a period of post–World War II economic growth and prosperity in most countries. Having had a decade to recover from the war, countries turned their attention to internal, social issues. This is when the United States created Medicare and Medicaid. During the 1980s, virtually every industrialized country found itself confronting rising health care costs and became convinced that there was no end in sight. This is when governments in other countries began taking greater control over their health care systems. For its part, the United States opted to increase the role of the private sector around this time in the expectation that competition would provide the most effective mechanism for addressing rising costs. Policy makers in other countries found some of the arrangements developed in the United States worth testing, use of DRGs to monitor hospital costs, for example. By the late 1990s, the United States began focusing on other mechanisms, namely new data collection measures and software designed to measure quality of care. Policy makers in other countries took an interest in these developments as well.[14]

It is fair to conclude that other countries support competition as long as it does not interfere with the basic health care plan that covers everyone in the country. It is interesting to see how competition looks when other countries embrace it, isn't it? Somehow it does not look much like it does in this country.

Can we, in turn, learn from the experiences of other countries? Perhaps. You might have noticed in reading this chapter that at least one of the mechanisms we created bears a strong similarity to arrangements European countries have had in place for a very long time. Consider that mutual benefit societies, created to provide help in cases of illness and disability, existed well before most countries began developing national health care systems. They were built on the idea that everyone would contribute to the community fund even though they would not necessarily benefit from it during any one year, perhaps not ever. Sounds a little like the basis of BC-BS and the Kaiser Permanente plan, doesn't it? Americans celebrated the founding of BC-BS, less so in the case of the Kaiser Permanente plan, as a totally new idea invented in the United States.

Americans tend toward xenophobia—we seem to have a strong need to reject what is foreign. Unlike the Europeans and Japanese, who have been importing ideas based on our experiments, we prefer to think that we are better off creating new mechanisms from scratch. And as we just noted, policy makers also like to relabel arrangements that have been around for quite a while and present what they are advocating as a brilliant new idea. Health policy makers keep introducing a steady stream of mechanisms, which they are prepared to discard when the mechanisms fail to deliver what was promised. Then, they simply go on to invent and reinvent some more. Winston Churchill's judgment of American ingenuity may be apropos here. He is said to have observed that Americans can be counted on to make the right decisions—after exhausting every other possible option.

QUESTIONS AND ISSUES TO THINK ABOUT

- The obvious question here is: What do you like and dislike about the health care systems in other countries?
- Are there any features of the health care systems created by other countries that would benefit the United States? That Americans would be willing to adopt?

8

HEALTH CARE REFORM: IS IT WORKING?

This chapter speaks to the question raised in the first chapter, namely, what is your assessment of the health care system in this country—is it so bad that the whole thing should be dumped or can it and should it be fixed? Now that you know a lot more about our health care arrangements and the changes that have been introduced over the past few years, have you come up with a different answer than the one you started with? Do you have views on what needs to be altered? Or have you concluded that it is all so overwhelming that you don't know where to start in advocating change? I can certainly understand if the last statement sums up your reaction. Nevertheless, the system will be undergoing change because there are enough interested parties willing to work very hard to see the changes they want enacted. We really can't avoid watching the system change—for better or worse.

So prepare yourself to plunge ahead and give more thought to evaluating the U.S. health care system. It might help to assess what has changed since the ACA was enacted. In evaluating whether the ACA is producing any positive changes, it is important to ask what you want it to accomplish. Accordingly, this chapter begins with a review of data on how well the law is working in seeking our primary health system goals—increasing access to care, achieving cost containment, and improving the quality of care. Keeping in mind that capturing this information is a matter of tracking a moving target, we will be looking at the information that is available at the time this is being written. I am very much aware of the fact that new information is coming out every day.

As I said in the first chapter, so far, the new information is updating what we already know. It is not reversing what we know. That, of course, may change.

This chapter also outlines the flaws in the health care system that the ACA has not fixed. The chapter also takes a closer look at the alternative that the authors of the ACA left on the table—the single payer plan—to see why proponents of the single payer plan think it would be an improvement over the system we have in place now.

WHAT THE ACA ACCOMPLISHED

Balancing Access and Cost

The first year during which the health marketplaces were operating saw the number of uninsured in the country drop by about 25 percent. The exact number is difficult to pin down. Quite a few highly respected private sector organizations (Rand Corporation, Urban Institute, the Commonwealth Fund, Kaiser Family Foundation, Gallup) and government agencies (CBO and HHS), conducted surveys and all came up with slightly different estimates. However, it is generally agreed that 8 to 10 million Americans enrolled in a private health insurance plan through the marketplaces in 2014, the first year during which enrollment in a health insurance plan was required. According to the White House, the total number of people enrolled as of 2015 was 16 million. Whether the percentage of uninsured will continue to drop in future years is difficult to determine because of unforeseen changes in the law, how various states deal with Medicaid expansion, and additional enrollments that will come when the small company employer mandate goes into effect.

When the ACA was being drafted, the Congressional Budget Office (CBO) projected that 32 million more people would be insured by 2017. The authors of the ACA expected 95 percent of Americans to be insured. The Supreme Court's decision to drop the Medicaid expansion mandate in 2012 caused the CBO to reduce its estimate to 26 million persons. Enrollment during the first enrollment period exceeded CBO projections. The enrollment numbers that were being reported led to vigorous arguments among politicians and various talking heads expounding their views in the public media about whether the higher number can be treated as an indicator of the law's success.

Policy analysts agree that persons who meet qualifications for Medicaid and who live in states that have chosen to expand Medicaid are the primary beneficiaries of the ACA. Enrollment in Medicaid during 2014 grew by 18.5 million in states that expanded Medicaid, in contrast to 5.7 million in states that did not. Other beneficiaries are persons under age twenty-six who obtained coverage under their parents' health insurance plans. Persons with pre-existing health conditions benefited but there is no count how many people fall into this category. How much others benefited varies a lot by age, gender, race/ethnicity, and state in which they reside.

The law did not achieve universal coverage, but there was no expectation that it would. In the end, the extent to which the law succeeded in increasing access to care is a judgment call. It depends on whom you ask.

Cost Containment

Before the law could go to Congress for a vote, the CBO and the Joint Commission on Taxation (JCT) were required to calculate budget implications. The 2009 estimate was that the ACA would cost $788 billion over the following ten years. The CMS estimate was far lower at $251 billion. The difference between the two estimates is due to the fact that the CMS included revenue that would be generated during the same period. Mind boggling as these numbers are, CBO/JCT cost estimates have been lowered every year since they were issued. The 2014 estimate for 2015 through 2024 was $104 billion lower than the previous year's projection. The CBO announced that no new estimates would be forthcoming because the ACA is undergoing so many changes.

How about the cost of health insurance to the enrollee? Costs have been increasing at the rate of 10 percent per year since the ACA was passed. That means that there has been no blanket increase in premiums since the ACA went into effect. However, there was and continues to be a tremendous amount of variation by state. There is no single explanation to account for the variation. The number of insurers participating in a state's insurance exchange does have an impact. States that have a single dominant insurer tend to have higher rates. We will get back to this point in chapter 9.

Focusing on the cost implications of extending Medicaid, the indications, based on government data, are that: "Medicaid provides access to health care services comparable to ESI [employer-sponsored insurance] at a significantly lower cost."[1]

To the extent that the law has succeeded in containing costs, no one section of the law can be credited more than another. The reduction in Medicare Advantage payments from an average of 14 percent to 2 percent is clearly expected to reduce costs, but there is no data on this yet. The Medicare "bundled payment" program has gotten a considerable amount of credit. The bundled payment covers treatment by a physician, care in the hospital, and post-hospital care—coverage that begins three days prior to hospitalization and spans thirty days post-hospitalization. The plan is not only expected to lower costs but to increase quality. The reduction in hospital payments for "never events" is already said to be reducing costs and increasing quality. HHS credits introduction of the Prevention and Public Health Fund (PPHF) for some of the savings. According to HHS, chronic illness accounts for seven out of every ten deaths and 75 percent of the nation's health care spending. Investing in prevention of chronic illness saves $5.60 for every $1.00 in spending.

Despite the evidence that has been accumulating, interpretations of the degree to which the ACA has produced cost containment have been restrained. It is clear that the percentage of the GDP allocated to health expenditures has been stable at 17.4 percent for the four years since passage of the ACA. The rise in costs has not been so low since the 1960s. Spending growth slowed over the past couple of years in most categories—in medical services, hospital care, Medicare, health insurance, and out-of-pocket spending. Cost increases occurred in Medicaid and retail pharmaceutical drugs.[2]

According to HHS, the ACA is saving money and improving care "by shifting attention from sickness and disease to wellness and prevention." Nevertheless, policy analysts have been cautious in their assessment of the extent of cost containment achieved by the ACA because all the factors that would have to be considered to arrive at a conclusive statement are so complex. What they end up saying involves a double negative—that it is unreasonable to argue that the ACA has had no cost containment impact.

Beyond that, even the loudest opponents of the ACA, who say that it has not succeeded in reining in spending on health care, are not willing to make explicit how they would go about cutting costs further other than getting government out of the picture entirely. The discussion is touchy because it hazards turning the focus on how the government does spend its money. To put this in perspective, consider the 2014 distribution of federal expenditures: 8 percent for Medicaid, 17 percent for Medicare, 24 percent for social security, and 33 percent for defense, leaving 18 percent for all other federal expenditures. It is enlightening to see where one's tax dollars are going, isn't it?

Quality

Another phrase that has become very popular over the last couple of years is "quality of care, not quantity of care." The statement is meant to convey the idea that the health care system in this country has been rewarding providers for doing more whether that results in a better *outcome* or not. Determining whether the ACA has had a positive effect on quality of care presents a problem for good reason—there is no consensus on a single measure of quality.

Given that increasing access to care was given so much prominence in how the ACA was initially presented, it is interesting to see how much attention the law devoted to improving quality of care. One of the most notable tools created by the ACA is the National Quality Strategy (NQS) under the auspices of the Agency for Healthcare Research and Quality (AHRQ). The organization was mandated to identify health care quality priorities. About 300 groups and individual experts came together to create tracking mechanisms and levers to accomplish the priorities they set. Participants who brought varying perspectives to the project say that the process was effective, the recommendations are fair, and the effort will bring needed reforms. The NQS released its first report in 2011.

A number of other entities created by or alongside the ACA have taken shape and begun to function such as the Patient-Centered Outcomes Research Institute (PCORI). This is a nonprofit organization designed to operate under the auspices of a multi-stakeholder board charged with identifying research priorities and conducting research that compares the clinical effectiveness of medical treatments.

The National Prevention, Health Promotion, and Public Health Council, comprised of twenty agencies and departments chaired by the Surgeon General, was established with the aim of coordinating prevention efforts. Along the same lines, a more concrete step intended to benefit people's health is the requirement that private health insurance cover preventive services; plus, the fact that copayment for preventive services under Medicare and Medicaid was eliminated.

Finally, the law requires chain restaurants and vending machine foods to have nutritional information for each item. And sun tanning salons were slapped with a 10 percent tax, in recognition that indoor tanning presents a serious risk of melanoma—cancer of the skin.

Evidence that the ACA has had an impact will take some time to collect because health improvements cannot be expected within a year or two. But there are a few studies to look at. For example, an AHRQ study found a 15 percent decline in hospital-acquired conditions from 2010 to 2013.[3] Which the agency said translated into $12 billion in savings. There is also evidence that screening rates increased, particularly for colon cancer; persons under the age of twenty-six have been more likely to report excellent health than they did previously; and, more young people have been taking advantage of newly covered mental health services.

A study specifically targeted to measure the impact of the effect of Medicaid expansion is noteworthy. A comparison between a number of adjacent states, which did or did not extend Medicaid, indicates that mortality rates decreased in the states that did extend Medicaid.[4]

Other organizations have concentrated their efforts on measuring the quality of the care linked to health plans. The National Committee for Quality Assurance (NCQA), which is a nonprofit organization, ranked 984 health plans using thirty-two clinical performance measures. It is interesting to see that the top ten plans are managed by nonprofit organizations. *Consumer Reports* publishes evaluations of doctors and hospitals based on measures it has developed. The most comprehensive evaluations of all doctors and all hospitals in the United States released in 2013 and 2014 by the CMS have only begun to be analyzed. The data sets are massive and not readily accessible to most people.

UNRESOLVED PROBLEMS

Much of what can be said about the access problems that continue to plague the U.S. health care system can be characterized as unevenness, inconsistency, unfairness, or disparity.

Access

The primary example of unevenness and inconsistency in access is that people whose income falls under 138 percent of poverty have no health care coverage in states that refused to expand Medicaid. Another example is the large variation in the premiums from one state to another that people enrolled in private health insurance must pay. Additionally, annual increases in premiums are not the same from state to state. Yet another blatant example of unevenness and unfairness occurs because there is no uniformity in the share of the premium employees are required to pay across employer-sponsored insurance plans. (This raises issues to which we return in chapter 9.)

There is growing concern about costs of health care services beyond insurance premiums. The least expensive health insurance plan, the Bronze plan, has the lowest premium but the highest deductible. The tax subsidy that is offered to persons with income up to 400 percent of poverty covers premiums but not copayments, deductibles, and other costs. Thus people who can afford the insurance policy may still not be able to afford health care services because of high out-of-pocket costs. The result is *underinsurance*.

While administrative cost, calculated as the medical-loss ratio, in the case of private insurance has been restricted to 15 percent, the administrative costs in one public insurance plan, Medicaid, have not been addressed. Critics regularly point out that the money spent determining whether a person is poor enough to qualify for Medicaid, that is, *means testing*, is money wasted. That the money would be better used to provide health care. More is wasted in cases when Medicaid enrollees are employed for a period of time then lose their jobs and are forced to go through the application process again, a process that may be repeated over and over again. As you recall from chapter 6, this is known as "churning."

Churning is not a term used to describe what happens in the private health insurance market. In that case, enrolling in a different plan is defined as a privilege enjoyed by consumers who can choose to shop for better coverage in the health marketplace. Indeed, Americans are being criticized for not shopping for a better plan from year to year. But enrolling and disenrolling from year to year in private insurance plans is tantamount to churning. On the insurance company side, it is an administrative cost that enters into medical-loss ratio calculations and the overall price of insurance plans.

Another issue that is just beginning to receive attention has to do with the variation in administrative capability and performance by states. Giving states responsibility for monitoring the operations of state health insurance marketplaces is intended to allow states the freedom to determine which health insurance organizations may participate in each state's health marketplace. The fact that each state must figure out how to set up its own administrative procedures, hire its own staff, and so on is being questioned by some. There is no data on how much this is adding to the country's health care expenditures. Consider why costs might increase. Not only is it costly to set up a department that will handle such matters, it is not necessarily efficient and effective for each state to build its own agency from scratch. What has become clear is that many states are poorly equipped to monitor the health markets. Some states do not have the funds; others are unwilling to devote the necessary funds; still others do not make the right choices in hiring qualified persons to accomplish these tasks.

As an aside, one of the first steps that corporations take after entering into corporate mergers is the elimination of duplicative administrative units. People are fired and money is saved when the administrative work carried out by companies involved in mergers is consolidated.

The 15 percent limit on administrative costs mandated by the ACA to manage private health care plans versus the 2 percent that it costs to run Medicare is difficult to justify. The argument presented by opponents of the ACA who say that Medicare amounts to a takeover of the health care system is not very convincing given that Medicare uses Medicare Administrative Contractors (MACs). It contracts with private insurance companies to process Medicare claims. Use of a competitive bidding process to arrive at negotiated contracts means that administrative costs are predictable rather than open ended.

"Unevenness" as Illustrated by the Dartmouth Atlas

The Dartmouth Atlas provides graphic illustrations of the extent of the inconsistency in the delivery in health care services across different regions in this country. The Atlas came into existence as a result of the early efforts of Dr. John Wennberg, who wanted to understand why there was so much variation in the numbers of people getting certain kinds of treatment in Vermont, where he was working at the time.[5] There was little explanation for the variation because the patients, all Vermont residents, were similar across all the variables that might explain different rates. He also did not think that doctors in one part of Vermont were greedy and doing more to make more money and that doctors in other communities were less greedy. So what is the explanation? In interviewing doctors he found that their practice patterns were shaped by their early training. They were simply doing things the way leading professors of medicine taught them to do things, to treat illness more aggressively or less aggressively. As you will recall, this came up in chapter 4, when we discussed why doctors became interested in specializing in the wake of World War II. Leading figures in the field, highly regarded medical professors, have a powerful influence on what constitutes first-rate medical care.

As an aside, if you are not convinced, you might be interested in hearing about a researcher who had doubts about doctors' selflessness. He devised a clever test. He checked to see whether doctors used the same tests and treatments on their own children. It turns out that in some cases they were just as aggressive or more aggressive. The researcher concluded that it was unlikely that they were doing that for the money.

This is not to deny the waywardness of doctors who accept "gifts" from pharmaceutical and medical device companies. As a matter of fact, a long debated piece of legislation, known as the Sunshine Act, was included in the ACA. It requires pharmaceutical companies and medical device manufactures to report payments and gifts to physicians and teaching hospitals and list their names. The CMS released its first report covering (only) the last five months of the year in September 2014. The report identifies $4.4 billion in payments.[6] No one disputes the fact that the companies make the payments in an effort to influence doctors and hospitals' choices of drugs and equipment. The companies get to write this off as a business expense. The companies recoup these expenditures by increasing the price of their products. Stopping the practice has been challenging because it is difficult to prove that the doctor is advocating a certain medication for the money as opposed to a real conviction that it works.

Getting back to the Dartmouth Atlas, it tracks procedural variations across the country and presents the illustrations on its web site. A number of researchers, doctors, epidemiologists, and others joined Wennberg in trying to determine the impact of varying treatments on outcomes. The results are eye opening! A number of excellent books written by his colleagues raise challenging questions. Gilbert Welch presents a powerful argument for doing less testing in his book *Overtested*.[7] He argues that preventive care is crucial, but that the tests often identify problems that might never result in illness. Once such indicators are found, more tests follow. Treatments follow too. All this obviously increases costs. The stress patients experience in worry about having a serious illness is incalculable. The fact that the high-tech testing equipment is there, the institution encourages doctors to use it, patients are quick to sue if the tests are not carried out, and the more tests doctors do, the more they are paid—all contribute to overtesting, according to Welch.

Other members of the group point out that testing people for possible health problems makes no sense if the person is too sick to tolerate the surgery necessary to address the problem. A surgical procedure performed on a fragile person may shorten the person's life, not extend it. Again, this carries unnecessary costs, especially when the testing and follow-up procedures take place in hospitals, which is where most health care dollars go, using high-tech equipment and all the personnel this requires. The costs related to keeping a person in a hospital bed who is brain-dead are particularly troubling and difficult to resolve. An excellent book that expands on all of these issues is Shannon Brownlee's *Overtreated*.[8] A compelling discussion of many of these issues is presented in a thought-provoking PBS video in which the authors mentioned here and others explore the relationship between money and medicine, titled *Money-Driven Medicine*.[9] What the work of researchers connected to this effort makes clear is that the explanation for variations in treatment patterns and the costs involved is far more complicated than greed on the part of doctors can explain.

Interest in the impact that variation in treatment has on costs is beginning to attract greater attention. A study of variation in hospital admissions that come through the emergency room is a case in point.[10] Conditions associated with low mortality vary most. Accordingly, the researchers suggest that standardizing ER hospitalization practices would produce greater efficiency and cost savings.

While the ACA does not target the problems revealed by the Dartmouth Atlas or other studies of variation in treatment, it is adjusting its reimbursement formula. It traditionally paid different rates by region of the country but is now reducing the rate paid to high-expenditure regions and increasing the rate in low-expenditure regions. The reimbursement formula does not attempt to take variations in quality into consideration because the formula for doing that would be too complicated. Consider the examples of variation reported by the AHRQ in 2006.[11] The District of Columbia ranked first for its low suicide rate and fifty-first for the highest colorectal cancer death rate; Kansas ranked third for its low HIV-related death rates but forty-eighth for death rates for patients who did not receive recommended care in the hospital; Oregon ranked first for the number of adults who received pneumonia vaccine, but forty-sixth for improving the health of home health patients. The AHRQ publishes a State Snapshots tool online. It does not attempt to explain why such variations exist, nor does it offer a solution.

Cost Containment

A report issued by the Organisation for Economic Co-operation and Development (OECD) offers a thorough analysis of the factors that explain why the United States spends so much on health care compared to other economically advanced countries.[12] It states that "A 2010 OECD study . . . found that the US price level of hospital services to be over 60% higher than the average of 12 other OECD countries in 2007." The report goes on to present a revealing picture of how much the United States differs in how it spends its health care dollars. It turns out that the United States, on average, invests in more technology but invests considerably less in numbers of doctors, doctor consultations, hospital beds, hospital discharges, and lengths of stay.

Although a considerable amount of evidence exists to indicate that national health care costs in the United States have not risen over the last few years and that the premium enrollees pay has remained stable, there is less known about the out-of-pocket expenditures. Although the ACA caps out-of-pocket expenditures at $6,350, there is little research to indicate how many people are finding out-of-pocket costs below this figure to be financially burdensome. This is where concern about underinsurance comes in. One of the few reports comes out of the *New York Times* series "Paying Till It Hurts." The *New York Times* in cooperation with CBS conducted a survey of 10,000 readers in 2014.[13] The results indicate that the percentage of respondents who said that "affording medical care" posed a hardship increased from 36 percent to 45 percent from 2013 to 2014. Out-of-pocket costs "went up a lot" according to 33 percent; "a little" according to 19 percent; and "stayed the same" for 39 percent; meaning that 52 percent reported spending more out-of-pocket than they felt comfortable spending over that period. There was little agreement on a solution. However, 80 percent said that doctors should discuss the cost or treatment.

As an aside, I want to point out that asking doctors to discuss treatment costs would be difficult to arrange because doctors don't have the information they need to provide accurate costs. Doctors in private practice can tell patients what they will charge for an office visit or a particular kind of treatment. Doctors who are salaried or work on a contractual basis may not know what the organization they are associated with charges for the full range of services, but they could probably find out. Getting the information on what the hospital will charge, what other doctors who consult or assist in surgeries will charge, what the organizations that read and report test results will charge, what pharmaceuticals the patient needs will cost—considered all together means that coming up with a number is pretty much impossible. Even if doctors could come up with some figures, those figures might not be accurate from one patient to another and from one period of time to another. Asking doctors to invest time in coming up with prices is just not a reasonable use of resources—the doctor could be doing something far more beneficial, namely providing health care services.

Here is another aside: some policy makers persist in arguing that doctors should inform themselves. This is where what I said in the first chapter about telling somebody what they should do becomes relevant.

Saying doctors should be doing this is clearly futile as a policy if there is
no mechanism for carrying it out, let alone having an incentive for doing
it. If it were possible to compile the information, which would certainly
require a lot of time to do, explaining it to patients would take even
more time. There has been little discussion about reimbursement for
time spent discussing costs with patients. What I find mystifying is that
those policy makers, who are so adamant about what doctors *should* do,
have shown far less interest in telling the parties that have the information what *they* should do, namely, make the information available.

Cost Containment and Quality

A number of explanations for high costs and questionable quality are
now widely accepted. As noted earlier, it is clear that having more high-
tech machines translates into more tests. It has also become clear that
more tests carried out in institutions that have a low volume of carrying
out those tests correlates with increased risk to the patient. Technicians
may not have enough experience to recognize that the machines are not
operating effectively. This is especially risky in the case of CT scanners,
which may emit excessive amounts of radiation. There is good evidence
to show that persons who perform a low number of procedures make
more errors than those who carry out more tests and become more
experienced. In other words, many machines in many institutions increases costs and lowers quality. (This obviously goes to the point discussed in the first chapter, that is, that many Americans believe that
having so many high-tech machines is what makes our system superior.)

Another widely shared conclusion has to do with the ratio of specialists to primary care practitioners in this country. Specialists do what
they are trained to do, carry out tests, do procedures, including surgical
procedures, just as the Dartmouth Atlas researchers found to be the
case. High-tech procedures and surgery are the most costly forms of
medical practice. To the extent that we are becoming concerned about
getting too many tests and too much surgery, then we should not be
educating so many practitioners to do this kind of work. As the policy
analysts with the Dartmouth Atlas are prone to say in reference to
specialists' practice patterns: "if the only tool you have is a hammer,
then everything looks like a nail." Why we have so many specialists, far
more than most economically advanced countries, is not hard to ex-

plain. Medical residents are not likely to choose family practice given that the incentive system directs more financial and other rewards to specialists. (While that was true right after World War II, as we discussed in chapter 4, the increase in number of specialists has accelerated tremendously since then, as have the rewards for entering into specialty practice.) Many high-prestige institutions have reduced or eliminated entirely family practice residencies. (It is not hard to understand why those institutions have concluded that there is little prestige in training family practitioners.) Patients self-refer to specialists because they are convinced that specialists offer superior care. In actuality, specialists do perform all those impressive procedures. But they do not provide preventive care or continuing care after the procedure. There is little disagreement about the fact that preventive care, when done well, does exactly that—it goes a long way in preventing patients from getting sick enough to require those expensive procedures. Preventive care is the province of primary care physicians.

Cost savings achieved by denying Medicaid is another misguided policy, according to many policy analysts. Denying people access to preventive and continuing care means that they will be sicker when they do seek care. And they will seek care in emergency rooms because they can't afford to see a doctor before they are seriously ill. Refusing to extend Medicaid, because it costs too much, makes no sense. It is short-sighted. Like raising the Medicare eligibility age that we discussed earlier, refusing to extend Medicaid just shifts costs. Hospitals end up paying for the care of uninsured patients and the federal government ends up reimbursing hospitals, at least in part. Private insurance companies raise their premiums in response to the high rates hospitals charge to make up for their losses. The people who are uninsured and too sick to work are not contributing to the economy by paying taxes, which would help cover health care costs. They may also end up qualifying for other forms of government assistance. And, of course, there is the incalculable cost of pain, suffering, and insecurity about the future that they have to bear. Yet cutting back on Medicaid is a policy that politically conservative politicians actively campaign on and impose if and when they can.

THE POLITICAL BATTLEFIELD AND THE ACA

It is hard to miss the fact that Democrats who are responsible for passage of the ACA do not appear to be wildly enthusiastic about it. They say something like, "it is a good first step but needs much improvement." As to the degree of opposition being registered by Republicans, there is no other explanation for the opposition other than political gain. The stance taken by Republicans certainly cannot be explained as a matter of financial judiciousness. States that refused to extend Medicaid rejected a substantial amount of federal funding, as I pointed out earlier in the case of the state of Illinois, which missed getting $270 million allocated for setting up a Health Exchange. It is not that the states that refused to extend Medicaid are opposed to federal funds in principle. Most states actively seek out federal funding for such projects as highway construction, support for military bases, prisons, and all kinds of other projects. The funds to support such proposals are generally lower than the funds that went with the Medicaid extension of the ACA. Critics also point out that the citizens of the states that rejected Medicaid paid taxes that ended up as funds that went to other states.

The interesting upshot of the decision to refuse to extend Medicaid is coming back to haunt the governors of the states that refused to do so. Insurance company executives and hospital administrators are now registering displeasure at losing the opportunity to benefit from the financial gains that increasing numbers of insurance enrollees and insured patients have produced in states that extended Medicaid. This is confirmed by the vast increase in the value of for-profit hospital corporate stock reported in the business pages. Health insurance company stock has achieved an unprecedented rise in value, which is attributable, in large part, to the fact that private insurance companies are handling Medicaid in states that did expand Medicaid. Accordingly, the hospital organizations and insurance companies that have been prevented from sharing in the financial boom are pressing state governments that refused to participate in Obamacare to reverse that decision. It will be interesting to see how this plays out—who will be the victors in this political battlefield—Republicans who opposed federal intervention in their state's affairs or Republicans who now have reason to welcome it.

Then there is the lawsuit, *King v. Burwell*, that the Supreme Court agreed to hear in the autumn of 2014. The litigants charged that the

ACA legislation, as it was worded, did not permit the federal government to support tax subsidies in health markets established by the federal government in states that did not set up their own health exchanges. The intent of the suit was to dismantle the ACA by defeating the core goal of the law. According to a Rand Corporation report, eliminating the subsidies would cause 11 million Americans to lose their health insurance and increase private insurance premiums by 43 percent.[14] The Supreme Court decision came down in June 2015. The Court upheld the law saying that the ruling reflected the intent of the law, which was to provide subsidies to enrollees in every state.

Republicans have also campaigned on the promise to overturn the 2.3 percent medical device tax imposed by the ACA. This is based on the argument that the tax is too high a price for doctors and dentists to pay for the devices they use. Most important, the tax eliminates jobs and is a detriment to job expansion. Many observers don't believe that the tax presents much of blow to the medical device companies that are making impressive profits. Quite a few outside observers point out that this is a minor charge to make as a criticism of the ACA.

There is no way to predict what other challenges to the law will be forthcoming. Republicans promise that they will not give up and will continue in their efforts to overturn the law. In the meantime, analysts in agencies such as the CBO say that provisions mandated by the law have already been embedded and are unlikely to be unraveled. Opponents of the law have not been discouraged.

Also true is the fact that public polls keep reporting, as we noted in chapter 2, that the effort to repeal the law continues to get popular support. How repealing the law would work is not clear. There is good evidence, confirmed by the CBO report just mentioned, that the majority of people do not want to see major parts of the law repealed. The 2011 Kaiser Family Foundation poll outlines what the public wants to see maintained: 85 percent approved closure of the Medicare doughnut hole; 79 percent approved subsidies for low and moderate income health insurance enrollees; 67 percent approved Medicaid expansion. The public also liked the components that had been put into effect earlier, such as young adults staying on their parents' plans and helping people who are at high risk of serious illness and previously uninsurable to obtain insurance.[15]

There is one more problem that has come into focus during the first few months of 2015, namely the challenge of calculating income tax returns. Dealing with the impact on tax returns of the tax benefits and subsidies the ACA provides for the first time around is sure to cause confusion. Judging by ads appearing in various media outlets, companies that offer income tax services are not upset; they are not unhappy.

THE SINGLE-PAYER ALTERNATIVE

While a very large number of Americans are undoubtedly tired of the debate surrounding passage of Obamacare and just want to have a health care system that works, stakeholders across the spectrum—politicians, policy experts, various interested organizations, including provider organizations, have reason to hope that their preferred solution will take effect. Curiously the basic hope is that the ACA will fail is widely shared across the political spectrum. What comes after that is where stakeholders part ways. On one side are those who want to see acknowledgment of the failure of government intervention in shaping the health care system. They want things to go back to where they were but with the private sector having a much bigger role. This faction is consistent in its position that the private sector is invariably more efficient than government. On the other side are those who believe that the patches that have been applied to the health care system over the years will cause it to collapse under its own weight. They maintain that enough people in this country will be ready to consider having a totally new system replace prevailing arrangements, a system more like the systems in other economically advanced countries. The survey discussed in the first chapter comparing the readiness of people in other countries to say that their health care systems should be rebuilt provides support for this interpretation. This contingent believes that the only rational thing to do is to institute a single payer system, a Medicare for everyone system.

This brings us to the fourth option, the single-payer plan, identified by the IOM for changing America's health care arrangements outlined in chapter 2. Discussion about this option has largely been overshadowed by the attention the ACA has been receiving. It is interesting to find that a 2009 *New York Times* poll, conducted before the ACA was enacted, found that 72 percent of Americans would have liked to see a "Medicare for all" type of plan instituted. [16]

Outline of the Single-Payer Plan

One of the most comprehensive summaries of the single-payer proposal is outlined by the Physicians' Working Group for Single-Payer National Health Insurance in a 2003 article in the *Journal of the American Medical Association*. [17] It is based on four principles:

1. insurance coverage should not be tied to employment
2. the right to choose a physician is fundamental
3. corporate profit has no place in caregiving
4. medical decisions should be determined by patients and doctors, not corporations or government bureaucrats.

The authors say that "The United States alone treats health care as a commodity distributed according to the ability to pay, rather than as a social service to be distributed according to medical need." [18] They argue that the advantages of providing universal access are obvious. Not only would people be healthier and more productive if they were assured that they could get health care when they needed it, they would not run up high costs resulting from delayed care. They maintain that eliminating private insurance would result in an immediate drop in health care expenditures because administrative costs would decline sharply.

They make the point that half of bankruptcies in this country are attributable to medical debt. In fact, when those going through bankruptcy are surveyed, 78 percent report medical debt. [19]

In a 2002 article, two of the founders of the Physicians Working Group for a Single-Payer National Health Plan argued that the government's current health care cost burden was being underestimated. Only the costs of direct government expenditures on Medicare, Medicaid, Veterans Administration, public health, and hospital subsidies were included in the calculations. They wanted to see the tax subsidies that government extends to employers for offering insurance and expenditures on public employee health insurance costs included. They maintain that this more accurate calculation would raise the government share of health care costs to 59.8 percent rather than the 45.3 percent being cited at that time.[20] By their calculations, the government's contribution must include "public funding" plus "tax financing." In short, they were advocating the elimination of this tax loss and using the resulting income to fund a national health care plan. Another way of looking at it is that the government is already shouldering nearly as great a proportion of the health care bill as countries that have national health programs.

A report issued by the IOM in 2004 extends the argument in favor of a single-payer plan. In calculating how much we spend compared to how much we lose by tolerating such a high level of uninsurance, the IOM reported that the economic losses stemming from lack of health insurance amounted to $65 to $130 billion a year due to higher disease and death rates among the uninsured.[21] Accordingly, the IOM concluded that there would be no increased cost resulting from extending health insurance to everyone. The IOM argues that the loss to the economy of people not working to their full capacity is higher than the estimated cost of providing insurance for all Americans.

Advocates of the single-payer plan regularly point out that the United States is an outlier in how much it spends on health care. It might be good to go back to when the United States began on the path that led it to become an outlier, to spend a greater proportion of its GDP on health care than other countries. Health insurance in other economically advanced countries began to expand in the wake of World War II just as it did in this country. What changed is that other countries reined in expenditures during the 1980s. Their governments began playing a bigger role in negotiating with all the parties involved—starting with bargaining with providers of health care services in their own countries and going on to negotiate with global companies, that is, pharmaceutical and medical device companies. This is when the United States increased its commitment to the idea that the private sector, more specifically the corporate sector, could get the job done more efficiently than government. The underlying rationale was that monetary incentives would motivate people to compete to provide the best services at the lowest prices, which those on Wall Street quickly translated into the memorable slogan "Greed Is Good."

There are those who argue that there is another reason to explain why health care costs increased over the decades preceding the Great

Recession of 2008. They say that Americans were readier to seek more health care because the economy was flourishing and people had more money to spend. That explanation works only if you follow it up by arguing that people in other economically advanced societies were not nearly as interested in seeking more health care services as their economies improved, which is certainly not true. What is incontrovertible is that the pace of the rise in health care costs in this country since the decade of the 1980s has been much greater than it has been in other countries. Furthermore, all those countries have been providing health care coverage for all their citizens all along.

You really can't miss seeing a pattern—we turned to the for-profit sector approach starting around 1980 because the country bought into the promise on the part of those who were telling us that for-profit organizations were capable of delivering health insurance and other health care goods and services more efficiently and effectively. The message just got louder as evidence continued to mount that costs were increasing at an unprecedented rate in this country. Costs did increase in other countries, but they did so at a much slower rate. Virtually all economically advanced countries managed to stabilize the rate of increase at around this time. We did not. It is not that all those countries rejected private sector participation. It is just that they have not been as ready to buy into the for-profit efficiency mantra to the same extent.

It is hard to understand why Americans are willing to accept projections presented by believers in for-profit solutions promising that costs will decline in the future if we just give market competition enough time. That is the story we have been hearing for decades and all the while costs have continued to rise, and at a faster pace than in all those other countries that have not chosen to use the for-profit approach.

Proponents of the single-payer plan have not given up. Bernie Sanders, the senator from Vermont, a single-payer advocate for many years, and Jim McDermott, a representative from Washington, introduced the American Health Security Act of 2013 in Congress using the slogan "health care from womb to tomb." Sanders does not mince words in explaining what the act aims to achieve. He says:

> Our system doesn't make economic sense and it certainly doesn't make moral sense. In a civilized society, every man, woman and child must be able to get the medical care they need regardless of income.[22]

If you want to hear more arguments pro and con this legislation there are a couple of videos you might like. One involves a debate on CNN with Senator Lindsey Graham, who has been quoted as saying that Obamacare "sucks."[23] Another reveals that some Republicans have reason to support the American Health Security Act.[24]

ANSWERING THE QUESTION: HOW WELL IS THE HEALTH SYSTEM WORKING?

We have now come full circle in examining the health care arrangements that exist in this country. We have much to be proud about. We get excellent medical care, at least those who can afford it, because they can afford to pay for generous, but expensive, health insurance plans and all the costs not covered by insurance plans. Researchers are making discoveries that are at the forefront of medicine. Patients are generally pleased with the care they are getting. But we have much to be dissatisfied about.

The scorecard on the "performance of the U.S. health care system" issued by the Commonwealth Fund in 2006 sums up the situation. Little has changed since that time except for the increase in the percentage of the GDP we devote to health care.

For the 16 percent of its gross domestic product that the United States spends on health care—double the median for industrialized nations—the United States gets some of the world's best hospitals and most specialized physicians. Despite spending all that money, however, the United States remains the only industrialized country in the world that does not guarantee universal coverage. It is not a leader in the adoption of health information technology, and it achieves neither the best outcomes nor the best quality of care compared to other nations. Wide variations within the United States in quality, access, and costs pull national averages down to well below benchmarks achieved by top-performing states, hospitals, or other providers.[25]

More alarming is the authors' conclusion:

> In sum, the scorecard indicates that the United States has broad opportunities to improve. It can do better, given the level of resources it has committed to health care. There is also much risk in failing to act: Cost and coverage vital signs are moving in the wrong

direction. To assure a healthy, productive nation, transformation of the health system is of great urgency.

Given that this was a statement made four years before passage of the ACA, the question we must ask ourselves is: has the country altered its course and gone in the right direction or is it still on the wrong course?

PILING ON YET ONE MORE REALLY BIG QUESTION

After devoting so much attention to the country's health care system, I want to introduce a brand-new question. Namely, do you think that a vastly improved health care system will, in turn, bring about a significant improvement in U.S. mortality and morbidity rates? Or are there other factors that explain why some people are sicker than other people? The Robert Wood Johnson Commission to Build a Healthier America answers this question. It outlines what it says is an "urgent agenda for improving America's health" because "access alone is not enough." [26]

Obviously, it is rather late in the discussion to raise this question. But it is important to address some of the basic questions that epidemiological data present us with. We know that mortality and morbidity patterns vary with race and ethnicity. Yet explaining why Hispanics, for example, have better mortality rates than whites is not so easy. We know that mortality and morbidity rates vary by income and education. Is that the explanation for the advantage that Hispanics enjoy or are there other factors involved? Are people sicker because they don't realize that they are behaving in ways that have negative effects on their health? How can anyone miss hearing about the behaviors that are certain to damage our health, such as smoking, drinking all those sugary drinks, or living life as a couch potato? In short, if you want to know what explains variation in life expectancy and lower morbidity rates then you have to deal with all the pieces in the puzzle. I take a closer look at all those variables in my book *Unequal Health*. [27]

That sounds like the discussion of the U.S. health care system has ended. But it doesn't mean we have run out of things to discuss, not by a long shot. Remember all the times I said we would be getting back to one point or another in chapter 9? It is now time to get back to those points.

9

PROVOCATIVE QUESTIONS AND CHALLENGING EXERCISES

Having examined the working parts of the health care system fairly thoroughly, we can now turn our attention to the question of how we might apply that knowledge. The challenge, as I see it, is defining the problem the questions raise. Doing something about the problems is another matter. That requires moving to another level of discourse and, more to the point, readiness to jump into the pitfalls inherent in the policy making process. I hope you are willing to try your hand at that. Having settled what we hope to accomplish here, let's begin.

THINKING ABOUT THE HHS

The first task that I suggest you embark on involves taking a closer look at the U.S. Department of Health and Human Services to get a grasp on the extent of its responsibilities. Here is where we start: go to the U.S. Department of Health and Human Services web site, HHS.gov; go to "about HHS"; then go to subtitle "HHS Organizations," then to "Operating Divisions." You will find the following eleven agencies listed under the HHS umbrella. Some of the agencies will be familiar, since we encountered them in earlier chapters.

Administration for Children and Family Services (AFC)
Administration for Community Living (ACL)
Agency for Healthcare Research and Quality (AHRQ)

Agency for Toxic Substances and Disease Registry (ATSDR)
Centers for Disease Control and Prevention (CDC)
Centers for Medicare and Medicaid Services (CMS)
Food and Drug Administration (FDA)
Health Resources and Services Administration (HRSA)
Indian Health Service (HIS)
National Institutes of Health (NIH)
Substance Abuse and Mental Health Services Administration
    (SAMHSA)

While you will probably want to wander around the individual agency sites to find what interests you, my suggestion is that you visit all the "learn more about the work of . . ." lines in each case. Consider what they do in light of their budgets. Find information on what the agencies say their goals are and what they say they have accomplished. Any thoughts on the respective agencies' achievements? How about the grant funds they distribute, are these well thought out?

There is a lot to look at and no way to comment on all of it. I am sure you can take on any part of this challenge that interests you perfectly well on your own, without my help. However, I want to share some of my reactions with you. In my estimation, all of the agencies do a good job of explaining what they do and how they do it. And they all have interesting stories to tell. The AHRQ, for example, is the agency that lists as one of its successes increasing patient safety through reduction of hospital-acquired infections, the drop in infections and the money this saves, which came up in earlier chapters. The NIH includes an interesting statement that documents the problems the researchers who receive grants from the agency have dealing with ups and downs in funding. The CDC outlines information on Ebola, which is of course a very serious topic. But the agency takes a break from that in presenting us with a game called "Solve the Outbreak." Speaking of serious issues, take a look at the budget information the FDA includes on its site. In the effort to reduce federal expenditures, Congress has mandated that corporations that require FDA approval pay a "user fee." That means that the FDA receives a significant proportion of its funding from the companies whose products it is evaluating. Does this strike you as a good way for the federal government to hold down expenditures or might it lead to predictable problems?

The provocative part of taking a closer look at the HHS is considering whether it would benefit us to see any of the responsibilities each of the agencies is charged with altered in some way. For example, would you be ready to argue the country would be better served by shifting responsibility for some functions into the private sector? How about the agencies' budgets, would you argue for reducing their budgets? Alternatively, increasing any of them? If your reaction is that there is no way you could answer such questions, I would point out to you that there are folks in Washington, DC, and elsewhere, who are sure that they know the answer. Might that cause you to wonder how well informed some of those folks are, and whether they have a good grasp of the work that HHS and the agencies it oversees are doing and how well those agencies are doing it?

A mixed batch of topics that I think could use more attention follow. This includes such issues as the "bundling" approach to reimbursement introduced by the CMS, malpractice, the number of doctors we need, who has the authority to write prescriptions, the role of advertising in the health care sector, and finally how well consumer-driven health is working. I would not be surprised if you find yourself getting into debates about some of these issues with people who have opinions, informed or not, on these topics.

"BUNDLING"

The basic question here is: Do you think this form of reimbursement is superior to fee-for-service? Remember, bundling involves giving providers, the doctors and hospitals working together to provide comprehensive care from prevention through to continuing care, a set amount of money. The value of this approach is being actively evaluated by researchers. What I think is interesting is to ask how this differs from previous prepaid care arrangements. How does it differ from the Kaiser Permanente plan and HMO arrangements? Is it comparable to putting a cap on health expenditures the way Canada does? Is bundling a matter of celebrating the "reinvention of the wheel" or is it really a new and better approach?

DOCTORS AND THE FACTORS THAT CONTRIBUTE TO THE COST OF MEDICAL CARE

As mentioned in chapter 4, funds to support five-year demonstration projects have been allocated by the ACA in an effort to provide an alternative to the current approach to malpractice, which some observers say has reached crisis proportions. The way malpractice is handled raises a number of questions. First, what about the cap on "pain and suffering" awards? What are the pros and cons of setting a cap of $250,000? Or $500,000, as is true in some states? Who benefits and who loses when there is a cap?

Second, apart from the "pain and suffering" part of the settlement, how do you feel about the fact that the courts deal with malpractice? Are the courts the best mechanism for judging whether malpractice actually took place? Do judges and juries have the competence to evaluate the work done by a doctor? The lawyers on both sides do rely on expert witnesses with medical training. It is worth taking a closer look at this practice. Appearing as a witness takes a lot of time, time away from a busy schedule. The experience can be unpleasant if the opposing lawyer wants to get aggressive about challenging the testimony. There are, however, doctors who are willing to take on this burden on a regular basis and be paid for it. Lawyers rely on these doctors to testify in a wide range of cases. Is that a good solution to the need for expert advice? Is there a better way to handle this? In fact, is the court the right place to determine whether the doctor made a mistake?

Third, that brings up the issue of what you want to achieve through malpractice suits. Do you want to ensure that the doctor is punished for the harm the doctor caused or to make sure the doctor does not cause such harm again? Does it matter whether the doctor engaged in behavior that resulted in harm due to negligence (caused by drug or alcohol abuse, for instance) or because the doctor was not using the latest evidence-based procedures or did not have sufficient training to carry out the medical or surgical procedure? If a doctor knowingly caused harm or caused it through negligence then the suit becomes a criminal case rather than a malpractice suit. Otherwise, the suit is settled via a payout. The malpractice insurance carrier pays. When you think about it, the financial penalty to the doctor who is at fault is insignificant. The insurance premium will go up for the doctor, but it will go up anyway, because other doctors were successfully sued for malpractice too, raising the cost of the insurance for all doctors. If the case rests on the fact that the doctor did not have sufficient knowledge to perform the tasks that resulted in harm to the patient, is a malpractice settlement a good way to address that? Is malpractice the best mechanism to ensure that the doctor will alter the way he or she handles the kind of problem that led to the suit the next time a patient presents the same symptoms?

The reputational impact may actually constitute a more serious punishment. There is justice in that. But can you be absolutely sure the malpractice suit was warranted and the damage to the doctor's reputation is merited?

Fourth, what about the contingency fee? Remember, other countries prohibit this practice. Is the contingency fee an arrangement that benefits patients who could not afford to sue otherwise? Or is it an arrangement that encourages patients to sue on the chance that they will benefit? Doctors say lawyers are primarily interested in drumming up business, not reducing the risk of harm to patients. What is your reaction to the two sides of this argument?

DOCTORS, HOW MANY THE COUNTRY NEEDS

Americans believe that a person should be able to opt for any career the person chooses assuming the person can meet the qualifications. It is the last part that invites some scrutiny. How these issues are handled in Canada informs this discussion.

Medical students pay for medical school tuition and all related expenses in the United States. However, Medicare supports residency training. If Medicare is paying for it, shouldn't Medicare have a say in the number of residencies it is willing to support? How about the kinds of specialty slots that it will make available? What is your reaction to having the government assume authority for determining both the number of physicians who enter practice and the distribution of medical specialties? What are the arguments pro and con government intervention in this instance? Who would you suggest participate in making such determinations, assuming there is agreement that Medicare will be given the authority to intervene?

A related question is: Should the government subsidize the cost of medical school? If doctors did not bring a huge amount of medical debt to their practice, would they charge less? One way to look at it is—the government will pay, it is just a question of whether the government pays before or after the fact, subsidizing medical education or in reimbursing doctors for the services they provide.

Some observers say (as they did when medical schools were first accredited) that medical education has become far less affordable than was true in the past, so that only the sons and daughters of higher-income families can afford a medical education. Is this a problem that is worth attending to? Would it benefit society to have medical education heavily subsidized to allow individuals from lower-income families enter medical school? What difference, if any, would that make?

Whether the government should be involved in monitoring the number of doctors who come down the pipeline is an issue because it involves how much the government spends on health care. Some policy analysts argue that there will not be enough doctors to go around because of the aging population, more people with health insurance, and so on. This leads to the question of what effect increasing the number of doctors will have on access, quality of care, and cost containment. The answer depends on which side of the very large fence one stands on. Those who are on the classical economic theory side tell us increasing the supply of doctors will produce a drop in the price of health care services as the supply-demand curve predicts. Those on the other side of the fence say that increasing the supply of doctors will cause them to increase the number of procedures they perform in order to compensate for any lost income that the increasing supply of doctors produces. And that this will increase costs rather than lower costs. The argument is about "supplier-induced demand." They also say that increasing the supply of specialists who perform the most expensive kinds of procedures will increase costs far more than increasing the supply of primary care practitioners. Which side of this enduring argument, and all related offshoots of the argument, do you find more convincing?

WHO IS LICENSED TO PRESCRIBE?

States not only issue the license to practice medicine, they determine the scope of practice. They specify what practitioners with different kinds of training are permitted to do. The list of practitioners who are licensed to prescribe or dispense medications is short—MDs, DOs, dentists, podiatrists, nurse practitioners, physician assistants, and EMTs. Other groups have been actively campaigning to gain the license to prescribe. Most recently it is psychologists. They have succeeded in gaining prescribing privileges in some states. Recently that happened in Illinois, the state in which I live. The event made me curious. Exactly who is it in the state that makes this determination? I discovered that the Public Health Committee constituted by the Illinois State Legislature made the decision. Let's not leave it there. I wanted to know more about this committee, which I must admit I had not heard about until this time. I discovered that it was composed of eight people, all political appointees. That was not altogether surprising. What was surprising is finding that none had health care related educational credentials and from what I could tell, any health care related experience. Should the people who make such decisions have such credentials? Any particular kinds of credentials? How public and transparent should the appointments process be? Would it better if the decision making process had involved health care experts or data of any sort? Or does suggesting any change in this arrangement amount to a lot of unnecessary fuss?

ADVERTISING

The only other economically advanced country, besides the United States, that permits advertising of health care products is New Zealand. So what is wrong with advertising? The answer is that it was traditionally considered undignified and unprofessional in this country up until the last decade or two. Just think about the advertising about all kinds of things you see on the Internet, on TV, on billboards, in newspapers, and all around us. Do you believe that the ads are meant to convey accurate information or are the ads meant to entice the buyer to purchase the product or service whether there is any need for it or not? It is more accurate to say that truth in advertising is a slogan and not a reality? Do you have a view on that?

Those who favor advertising for health care products and services say that it informs patients and enables them to make better choices. How well does advertising accomplish that? Are the best doctors and hospitals putting their names out there? Is there any way to know that? Who makes the decision to do the advertising? Where is the money to pay for the ads coming from?

Pharmaceutical (pharma for short) advertising evokes the most criticism on the part of policy analysts. The market is saturated with pharma ads. We have all been encouraged to "ask your doctor" because it is sure to do great things for us. (The FDA regulations specify that ads using this exact phrase are permissible.) Have you seen the same ads I have—ads that are somewhat vague about the medical problem that the drug is supposed to address showing a person in glowing health skipping through a field of spring flowers and grass to illustrate the effect? Doctors complain about all the ads advising patients to ask their doctors. Doctors say that it takes time to convince patients that the drugs that they are certain will do so much good are not indicated for the patient's problem for various reasons. In many cases, doctors argue that making some behavioral changes would be far more beneficial than taking drugs. It seems that most of us would rather take a pill than change our diets or get more exercise. Doctors admit that some patients are so insistent that they give the patient the medicine to put a stop to the argument even if they think it will do no good but will not do harm. Of course, all those patented medicines and over-the-counter medicines Americans are convinced will produce wonderful results are adding tremendously to our health care bill.

Far more troubling is the fact that pharmaceutical companies are businesses that are under pressure to increase profits. Evidence of the degree to which they are pressured to do that can be found on the business pages rather than the front pages of newspapers. Business pages also report the staggering amounts of money pharmaceutical companies pay out to settle suits charging them with fraud for neglecting to report dangerous side effects of drugs. The companies invariably admit fault and settle out of court to avoid having to reveal the results of research and testing carried out prior to release of the drugs. If you are interested in this issue, I recommend Marcia Angell's *The Truth About the Drug Companies*.[1] What Angell documents is shocking.

The money paid out in the settlements, reported regularly by business media, is factored into the price of the drugs the company sells. However, given that this is the second most profitable industry in the country (after petroleum), efforts to look more closely at pharmaceutical industry operations means taking on Wall Street. This presents policy makers with an inconvenient and troublesome obstacle. What are your views on the whole range of issues related to this vexing problem?

Policy analysts are not reluctant to call attention to the fact that the cost of pharmaceuticals is far lower in other countries. The governmental entities in charge of health care systems in other economically advanced countries bargain with pharmaceutical companies for lower prices. Countries a lot smaller than the United States still constitute enormous markets and are able to negotiate lower prices. Medicare legislation regarding the operations of Medicare Part D specifically prohibits the U.S. government from bargaining over the price of pharmaceuticals. The argument is that this would interfere with commerce. However, pharma is a global industry, meaning that other countries have a commercial interest in pharma profitability as well. That does not stop them from negotiating over the prices they are willing to pay for pharmaceuticals. Again, what are your views? Would giving the U.S. government the right to bargain over pharmaceutical prices result in too much government interference?

CONSUMER-DRIVEN HEALTH CARE SYSTEM

We now come to the core issue in assessing our health care arrangements. The basic question is: Do you consider yourself to be a knowledgeable consumer of health care services and products or do you consider yourself to be a patient who is dependent on a doctor's diagnosis and the treatment the doctor recommends?

We have been circling around this question throughout the book and referring, here and there, to the fundamental argument involved. The theoretical foundation for arguing in favor of a consumer-driven health care system is that health care services and products are no different than other products and services traded in the market. As health care consumers we get the products and services we demand. That in turn has the effect of increasing the supply of those products and services. The providers of those products and services are then forced to reduce the price of their offerings, which will benefit us all. As is apparent, these are the premises that came up in the discussion on medical and pharmaceutical advertising, the number of doctors the society needs, and the role of private insurance companies, to name just a few of the topics we have considered in this context.

In order to accept the contention that consumers are driving the health care market, one must first grant the assertion that it functions like markets for other goods and services. One must accept the idea that the market permits free choice among the products and services that best meet our preferences and best serve our needs. Health insurance marketplaces stand at the heart of this argument. The marketplaces bring a large number of health plans together in one place so that we can compare the offerings. The central idea is—a person can choose the health plan the person wants based on quality and price.

There are a number of glitches in this proposition. One of the glitches has to do with the number of health insurers participating in a state's marketplace. Remember that classical economic theory tells that a critical characteristic of the markets that work well to control price is participation by many buyers and many sellers. This is the primary mechanism that causes suppliers to compete with each other, to lower prices in order to attract buyers. However, if competition depends on the participation of many sellers, what happens to competition if there are many buyers but a very small number of sellers? The answer is obvious.[2] The GAO looked into this question. It analyzed insurance market concentration over the four-year period following passage of the ACA. It reports the following: "the three largest insurers had at least 80 percent of the total enrollment in at least thirty-seven states. In more than half of these states, a single insurer had more than half of the total enrollees."[3]

States are under no obligation to release enrollment data, which makes it difficult to carry out a more detailed examination of local markets within states. However, there is some evidence to indicate that insurers are engaging in "cherry picking" the regions of the state they want to operate in—the population they wish to enroll and the provider networks they want to work with. In locations they deem to be less profitable they do not compete for enrollees. Instead, they offer fewer plans and plans for which they charge higher premiums. This is the interpretation being offered by analysts for the variation in health insurance policy prices in the small number of states where the variation in regional rates have been tracked.

Given that the health insurance market is operating this way, saying that people are buying plans that reflect their preferences based on an assessment of cost and quality looks like a stretch. Arguing that the market is consumer-driven looks like an even bigger stretch. If there are many buyers and a very small number of sellers, might it be more accurate to say that the sellers are sorting buyers out based on what they can afford rather than what they might prefer? Who would prefer to buy a plan that carries high out of pocket costs if they could have a plan with low out of pocket costs? Yes, that is the way markets work—if you cannot afford the expensive product, you just have to settle for the cheaper product. That raises a very charged and controversial question, namely, is the market, as it is operating, the best way to allocate health insurance? Critics of the health care arrangements in this country answer this question by saying that access to health care should be a right, not a privilege. Where do you stand with regard to that statement?

There is much more to this argument. Judging by media reports, the problem is not that health insurance markets are not working. It is that we, as consumers, are failing to shop for the best price. We are not playing the role we have been assigned. We should be pressing insurance companies to lower their prices and we are not doing a good job of it.

That assessment draws attention to another glitch in the consumer-driven health care system argument. Employees whose employers offer health insurance are not in a position to choose a health care plan based on quality and price. Their employers restrict that choice. The assessment of the consumer-driven health proposition by one well-known and highly regarded economist is worth hearing. In his June 7, 2013, *New York Times* blog, Uwe Reinhardt tells us that he made the following statement at a gathering of top executives at the Business Council in the early 1990s: "If you want to find the culprit behind the health care cost explosion in the U.S. go to the bathroom and look in the mirror." In his view, employers in this country "have become the sloppiest purchasers of health care anywhere in the world." They offer employer-sponsored health insurance because of the tax advantage the company gets rather than the benefit it provides to employees. The fact that employees lose insurance coverage when they lose the job is added evidence of how dysfunctional this arrangement is, in his view.

Another particularly astute health economist, Robert Evans, makes a crucial observation that speaks to the consumer-driven system conceptualization, one that is obvious once you hear it. He points out that people are not likely to be as eager to shop for health insurance plans as they are for most other consumer products and services.[4] The motivation is just not there to learn about and shop for an insurance plan. To paraphrase what he says, people are not interested in scoring a great health insurance policy. They are interested in good health.

How about our role in acting as informed consumers in choosing the doctor and hospital we want? We are regularly reproached for not informing ourselves about their quality and prices. Of course, the insurance plan we sign up for, or our employer signed us up for, may mean that we have little choice about the doctors and hospitals we can select. If the policy does not restrict choice of doctors and hospitals, that still does not mean that we are in a position to choose the best doctor or the best hospital. Proponents of the consumer-driven approach have not had much to say about the fact that consumers have very little information on quality to enable them to buy an insurance plan based on quality and price. However, that has changed. As noted in chapter 4, we are now being loaded down with information. After all, the government has presented us with information on every doctor and every hospital. The difficulty is that the data sets are daunting and not accessible to the average person. But there are other sources of information—the glossy special sections of newspapers, billboards, and so on—which we have already discussed, that tell us about how great a particular group of doctors and/or hospital is. That is, of course, the kind of information that markets in all sectors of the economy, not just the health sector, are ready to present.

We may be doing a slightly better job of shopping for pharmaceuticals because we can at least get information on prices if not quality. However, most of us are probably not calling every pharmacy in the city to check the price of each of our prescriptions and doing so regularly to make sure that the prices have not changed. It is true that new web sites are appearing that provide us with price information. Getting information on quality is far more complicated. Determining whether drugs will do what they are meant to do is difficult for a number of reasons, including the reason we mentioned earlier in the chapter when we discussed pharma advertising. Beyond that, individuals may react to drugs differently depending on what other health conditions they have and what other drugs they are taking. The correct dosage may require some time to establish. There may be side effects that cause new problems, and so on.

So where do we end up in considering this issue? Would you say that getting the information on doctors, hospitals, and drugs is not really difficult given all the sources of information that the Internet provides? Would you say that consumers could be doing a lot more to inform themselves about health care products and services?

Or would you argue that taking the role of a health care consumer is not easy? It is time consuming. If one cannot readily get information on price and quality, then being an informed consumer is a tough assignment. As we have already said, we can see health care sector organizations acting like all organizations that present their offerings in the market. They are spending dollars trying to entice us to buy what they offer. Hospitals are installing waterfalls in their lobbies, telling us that these have a relaxing influence on patients who are stressed. They are building suites that have all the amenities you would expect to find at the Hyatt. And it is true that consumers register high levels of satisfaction with such amenities. Doctors try to set up offices in glamorous buildings to show that they are able to attract the most lucrative patients. Some might say that this means that the consumer-driven health care system is working to provide what the American health care consumer wants, whether one approves of these choices or not.

Others might say that all the attention being devoted to amenities would not be bad if people who wanted them were willing to shell out the extra money to get them. However, having the whole health care system being responsive to these consumer preferences has the effect of increasing the price of health care without medical benefit. Whether consumers have been influenced to regard such amenities as indicators of quality and that is why they are registering those preferences is an assessment that would be interesting to explore. Any thoughts on that?

There is one more part to the argument that proponents of the consumer-driven market emphasize that deserves attention, one with which Americans are very familiar, namely, that private sector organizations are invariably more efficient than government agencies. The argument is especially heated when it comes to health insurance. The premise that the government is inefficient does, however, overlook the fact that the private health insurance industry is being heavily subsidized by the government. The tax benefits and out of pocket subsidies government is paying to make insurance plans more affordable are only making a temporary stop in the wallets of consumers before going into the coffers of private insurance companies. If the private sector is more efficient than government, what explains why the government is shouldering the transaction costs (economic speak for administrative costs in this case) produced by a consumer-driven health care system? A bolder version of this question is: Can the private sector make health care services and products available to everyone in the country without being subsidized by the government?

As to controlling transaction costs, the ACA has instituted a limit on the medical-loss ratio. However, doesn't the fact that this figure has been at least seven times higher than the costs of administering Medicare make the claim that the private sector is more efficient questionable?

Where do you end up at the close of the discussion on consumer-driven health? Is it accurate to say that our health care system is being shaped by consumer demand? Is the consumer-driven market working to bring us the health care arrangements we want? That we need? How much confidence are you willing to invest in consumers' ability to evaluate price and quality? Is the health insurance market's dependence on negotiators or health advocates to make it consumer friendly consistent with the powerful image that the consumer-driven label is meant to convey? Is blaming patients for failing to act as good consumers enough to motivate patients to take a more aggressive role and turn themselves into informed consumers? I expect that I have left out a number of questions that you might prefer to consider.

IF NOT A CONSUMER-DRIVEN MARKET, THEN WHAT?

I am not about to present you with a dazzling answer to the question I have just raised. Instead, I return to the earlier discussion on other economically advanced countries because they are clearly achieving better results. They treat people as patients rather than consumers. They use a variety of mechanisms to ensure that patients receive high-quality health care goods and services at a lower price than we are paying. I do not suggest that we adopt any one country's system. I am suggesting that there are things we could learn from other countries. It is also true that quite a few communities in this country have instituted arrangements that achieve high-quality care and cost savings. While it is important to acknowledge the significance of what those communities have achieved, it is also important to admit that those achievements benefit a small number of Americans.

We end as we began. I leave you with the question of whether we could do a better job of delivering health care in this country than we are doing now, and the even more challenging question of what you think would help achieve that goal.

NOTES

1. THE HEALTH CARE SYSTEM

1. "Comparisons: Life Expectancy at Birth," in *The World Factbook* (Washington, DC: Central Intelligence Agency), https://www.cia.gov/library/publications/the-world-factbook/rankorder/2102rank.html.
2. Commonwealth Fund, "International Profiles of Health Care Systems," 2013.
3. "GDP (Official Exchange Rate)," in *The World Factbook*, https://www.cia.gov/library/publications/the-world-factbook/fields/2195.html.

2. OPINIONS ON HEALTH CARE REFORM

1. Kaiser Family Foundation, "Kaiser Health Policy Tracking Poll," http://kff.org/health-reform/poll-finding/kaiser-health-tracking-poll-april-2015/.
2. Mira Norton, Liz Hamel, and Mollyann Brodie, "Assessing Americans' Familiarity with Health Insurance Terms and Concepts, Quiz," Kaiser Family Foundation, November 11, 2014.
3. "Jimmy Kimmel on Obamacare vs. the Affordable Care Act," YouTube video, October 1, 2013, https://www.youtube.com/watch?v=sx2scvIFGjE.
4. CNN Opinion Research Corporation, "CNN/Opinion Research Poll," December 16–20, 2009, http://politicalticker.blogs.cnn.com/2009/12/21/cnnopinion-research-poll-december-16-20-2009/.
5. Jacob Hacker and Paul Pierson, *Winner-Take-All Politics: How Washington Made the Rich Richer—And Turned Its Back on the Middle Class* (New York: Simon and Schuster, 2010), 109.

6. Kaiser Family Foundation, "Kaiser Public Opinion Spotlight: Health Care and Elections," December 2014, online at http://www.kff.org/spotlight.

7. Kaiser Family Foundation, "Kaiser Tracking Poll, Public Opinion on Health Care Issues," May 21, 2010, http://www.kff.org/kaiserpolls/trackingpoll.cfm.

8. Gallup, "Confidence in Institutions," January 5, 2014, http://www.gallup.com/poll/1597/confidence-institutions.aspx.

9. Tom Smith and Jaesok Son, "Trends in Public Attitudes About Confidence in Institutions. General Social Survey 2012," Final Report of the NORC, May 2013.

10. Thomas Piketty, *Capital in the Twenty-First Century* (Cambridge, MA: Belknap Press of Harvard University Press, 2014); Thomas Piketty and Emmanuel Saez, "Income Inequality in the United States, 1913–1998," *Quarterly Journal of Economics* 118 (February 2003): 1–39 (for update tables and figures, see http://elsa.berkeley.edu/~saez/).

11. Robert Reich, "Foreword," in Richard Wilkinson and Kate Pickett, *The Spirit Level: Why Greater Equality Makes Societies Stronger* (New York: Bloomsbury Press, 2010), vi.

12. Bureau of Labor Statistics, *The Consumer Price Index: Concepts and Content over the Years* (Washington, DC: U.S. Department of Labor, 1978).

13. Robert J. Blendon and John M. Benson, "Americans' Views on Health Policy: A Fifty-Year Historical Perspective," *Health Affairs* 20 (March 2001): 33–46.

14. U.S. Department of Health and Human Services, "The 2011 HHS Poverty Guidelines," http://aspe.hhs.gov/poverty/11poverty.shtml.

15. Blendon and Benson, "Americans' Views," 34.

16. Blendon and Benson, "Americans' Views," 34–35.

17. For an insider's assessment of the change in tactics used by the health insurance industry regarding the health care reform debate prior to passage of health care reform legislation, see Wendell Potter, *Deadly Spin: An Insurance Company Insider Speaks Out on How Corporate PR Is Killing Health Care and Deceiving Americans* (New York: Bloomsbury Press, 2010).

18. Institute of Medicine, *Insuring America's Health: Principles and Recommendations* (Washington, DC: National Academies Press, 2004), 155.

3. HOSPITALS AND OTHER
HEALTH CARE ORGANIZATIONS

1. Anne Pfuntner, Lauren Weir, and Claudia Steiner, "Costs for Hospital Stays in the United States, 2011," Healthcare Cost and Utilization Project,

Agency for Healthcare Research and Quality, Washington, DC, December 2013.

2. E. H. L. Corwin, *The American Hospital* (New York: Commonwealth Fund, 1946).

3. "Hospital Service in the United States," *Journal of the American Medical Association* 90 (April 3, 1928): 1009.

4. CDC Fact Sheet, "Hospital Utilization (in nonfederal short-stay hospitals)," http://www.cdc.gov/nchs/fastats/hospital.htm.

5. "Uninsured Hospital Stays, 2008," Statistical Brief #108, Healthcare Cost and Utilization Project, Agency for Healthcare Research and Quality, Rockville, MD, April 2011, http://www.hcup-us.ahrq.gov/reports/statbriefs/sb108.pdf.

6. Maggie Mahar, *Money-Driven Medicine: The Real Reason Health Care Costs So Much* (New York: HarperCollins, 2006).

7. "CMS's Special Focus Facility Methodology Should Better Target the Most Poorly Performing Homes Which Tend to Be Chain Affiliated and For-Profit," GAO-09-689 (Washington, DC: United States Government Accountability Office, August 2009).

8. David Classen, Roger Resar, Frances Griffin, Frank Federico, Terri Frankel, Nancy Kimmel, John C. Whittington, Allan Frankel, Andrew Seger, and Brent C. James, "'Global Trigger Tool' Shows That Adverse Events in Hospitals May Be Ten Times Greater Than Previously Measured," *Health Affairs* 30 (April 2011): 581–89.

9. Kevin O'Reilly, "In ORs, 'Never Events' Occur 80 Times a Week," *American Medical News* 56 (January 28, 2013): 1, 4.

10. Jill Van Den Bos, Karan Rustagi, Travis Gray, Michael Halford, Eva Ziemkiewicz, and Jonathan Shreve, "The $17.1 Billion Problem: The Annual Cost of Measurable Medical Errors," *Health Affairs* 30 (April 2011): 596–603.

11. See the entire April 2011 issue of *Health Affairs*, titled "Gaps in Health Care Quality Persist."

12. Agency for Healthcare Research and Quality, "10 Patient Safety Tips of Hospitals," Publication #10-M008.

4. HEALTH CARE OCCUPATIONS

1. Howard Becker, Blanche Geer, Everett C. Hughes, and Anselm L. Strauss, *Boys in White: Student Culture in Medical School* (Chicago: University of Chicago Press, 1961), 419–33; Robert K. Merton, George G. Reader, and Patricia L. Kendall, eds., *The Student-Physician: Introductory Studies in*

the Sociology of Medical Education (Cambridge, MA: Harvard University Press, 1957), 295–96.

2. Committee on Quality of Health Care in America, Institute of Medicine, Linda T. Kohn, Janet H. Corrigan, and Molla S. Donaldson, eds., *To Err Is Human: Building a Safer Health System* (Washington, DC: National Academy Press, 1999), 26.

3. Michelle M. Mello, Amitabh Chandra, Atul A. Gawande, and David M. Studdert, "National Costs of the Medical Liability System," *Health Affairs* 29 (September 2010): 1569–77.

4. Paul Starr, *The Social Transformation of American Medicine* (New York: Basic Books, 1982), 112–23.

5. Emily Berry, "Insurers Mishandle 1 in 5 Claims, AMA Finds," *American Medical News* 54 (July, 2011): 1, 4; Lawrence Casalino, Sean Nicholson, David Gans, Terry Hammons, Dante Morra, Theodore Karrison, and Wendy Levinson, "What Does It Cost Physician Practices to Interact with Health Insurance Plans?" *Health Affairs* 28 (2009): w533–w543.

6. Grace Budrys, *When Doctors Join Unions* (Ithaca, NY: Cornell University Press, 1997).

7. Linda Aiken, Sean Clarke, Robyn Cheung, Douglas Sloane, and Jeffrey Silber, "Educational Levels of Hospital Nurses and Surgical Patient Mortality," *Journal of the American Medical Association* 290 (September 24, 2003): 1617–23; Linda McGillis Hall, Diane Doran, G. Ross Baker, George Pink, Souraya Sidani, Linda O'Brien-Pallas, and Gail Donner, "Nurse Staffing Models as Predictors of Patient Outcomes," *Medical Care* 41 (September 2003): 1096–109; Julie Sochalski, "Is More Better?: The Relationship Between Nurse Staffing and the Quality of Nursing Care in Hospitals," *Medical Care* 42 (February 2004): II-67–II-73; Jack Needleman, Peter Buerhaus, Soeren Nattke, Maureen Stewart, and Katya Zelevinsky, "Nurse-Staffing Levels and the Quality of Care in Hospitals," *New England Journal of Medicine* 346 (May 30, 2002): 1715–22; Kevin Grumbach, Michael Ash, Jean Ann Seago, and Janet Coffman, "Measuring Shortages of Hospital Nurses: How Do You Know a Hospital with a Nursing Shortage When You See One?" *Medical Care Research and Review* 58 (December 2001): 387–403.

5. PRIVATE HEALTH INSURANCE

1. Sylvia A. Law, *Blue Cross: What Went Wrong?* (New Haven, CT: Yale University Press, 1974), 6–12.

2. Rosemary Stevens, *In Sickness and in Wealth* (New York: Basic Books, 1989), 259.

3. Bruce Japsen, "Illinois Blues Balk at Go-Public Stampede," *Chicago Tribune*, June 10, 1999, 1, 4.

4. Gail Jensen, Michael Morrisey, Shannon Gaffney, and Derek Liston, "The New Dominance of Managed Care: Insurance Trends in the 1990s," *Health Affairs* 16 (January/February 1997): 125–36.

5. "Persons Enrolled in Health Maintenance Organizations (HMOs) by Geographic Region and State: United States, Selected Years 1980–2002," Report by the U.S. Department of Health and Human Services, Public Health Service, 2003, table 150.

6. Mark Hall and Christopher Conover, "The Impact of Blue Cross Conversions on Accessibility, Affordability, and the Public Interest," *Milbank Quarterly* 81 (2003): 509–42.

7. Robert Kazel, "Union Seeks to Limit Aetna Execs' Pay," *American Medical News* (April 12, 2004): 20.

8. Emily Berry, "Profits Keep Rolling In for Big Insurers Despite Reform," *American Medical News* (February 21, 2011): 32–33.

9. "State-Level Trends in Employer-Sponsored Health Insurance, A State-by-State Analysis," Robert Wood Johnson Foundation Report, April, 2013, http://www.rwjf.org/content/dam/farm/reports/reports/2013/rwjf405434.

10. Table 135, "Private Health Insurance Coverage among Persons Under 65 Years of Age, by Selected Characteristics: United States, Selected Years 1984–2009," *Health, United States, 2010: With Special Feature on Death and Dying* (Hyattsville, MD: National Center for Health Statistics, 2011), http://www.cdc.gov/nchs/data/hus/2010/135.pdf.

11. Donna Dubinsky, "Money Won't Buy You Health Insurance," *New York Times*, February 20, 2011, 10.

12. Sara Collins, Michelle Doty, Ruth Robertson, and Tracy Garber, "Help on the Horizon: How the Recession Has Left Millions of Workers Without Health Insurance, and How Health Reform Will Bring Relief—Findings from the Commonwealth Fund Biennial Health Insurance Survey of 2010," March 16, 2011, http://www.commonwealthfund.org/publications/fund-reports/2011/mar/help-on-the-horizon.

6. PUBLIC HEALTH INSURANCE

1. "Medicare: Medicare Advantage Fact Sheet," Henry J. Kaiser Family Foundation and Health Research & Educational Trust, March 2004, http://www.kff.org/Medicare/upload/Medicare-Advantage-Fact-Sheet.pdf.

2. Marsha Gold, "Medicare's Private Plans: A Report Card on Medicare Advantage," *Health Affairs* 28 (January/February 2009): w41–w54; Kim Bailey,

"Whose Advantage? Billions in Windfall Payments Go to Private Medicare Plans," Families USA Special Report, June 2007, http://www.familiesusa.org/assets/pdfs/Medicare-private-plans.pdf, 4.

3. Robert Pear and Edmund Andrews, "White House Says Congressional Estimate of New Medicare Costs Was Too Low," *New York Times*, February 2, 2004, http://kff.org/Medicare/fact-sheet/Medicare-spending-and-financing-fact-sheet/, A14.

4. Kaiser Family Foundation, "The Facts on Medicare Spending and Financing," July 28, 2014, http://kff.org/Medicare/fact-sheet/Medicare-spending-and-financing-fact-sheet/; "PDP-Facts: 2015 Medicare Part D Statistics Region (State) and National," http://www.q1Medicare.com/PartD-MedicarePartDPlanStatisticsState.php.

5. Lynn Etheredge and Judith Moore, "A New Medicaid Program," *Health Affairs* (August 27, 2003), http://content.healthaffairs.org/content/early/2003/08/27/hlthaff.w3.426/suppl/DC1.

6. National Clearinghouse for Long-Term Care Information, U.S. Department of Health and Human Services, http://www.longtermcare.gov.

7. Joel Finkelstein, "Millions Have Health Coverage Gaps—Commonwealth Fund Study," *American Medical News* (December 1, 2003): 10–11.

8. "Medicaid and CHIP Participation Rates," InsureKidsNow.gov, http://insurekidsnow.gov/professionals/report/index.html.

9. "Raising the Age of Medicare Eligibility: A Fresh Look Following Implementation of Health Reform," Henry J. Kaiser Family Foundation Program on Medicare Policy, publication number 8169, March 29, 2011, online at http://www.kff.org/Medicare/upload/8169.pdf.

7. THE HEALTH CARE SYSTEMS IN
OTHER COUNTRIES

1. Carolyn Hughes Tuohy, "Dynamics of a Changing Health Sphere: The United States, Britain, and Canada," *Health Affairs* 18 (May/June 1999): 129.

2. Odin Anderson, *Health Care: Can There Be Equity? The United States, Sweden, and England* (New York: Wiley-Interscience, 1972).

3. Rachael Jolley, ed., "State of the Nation: Where Is Bittersweet Britain Heading? *British Future* (January 2013): 25.

4. Rudolf Klein, "Britain's National Health Service Revisited," *New England Journal of Medicine* 350 (February 26, 2004): 937–42; Peter Smith and Nick York, "Quality Incentives: The Case of U.K. General Practitioners," *Health Affairs* 23 (May/June 2004): 112–18; Simon Stevens, "Reform Strategies for the English NHS," *Health Affairs* 23 (May/June 2004): 37–44.

5. Reinhard Busse and Juliane Stahl, "Integrated Care Experiences and Outcomes In Germany, The Netherlands, and England," *Health Affairs* 33 (September 2014): 1549–58.

6. John Iglehart, "Germany's Health Care System (First of Two Parts)," *New England Journal of Medicine* 324 (February 14, 1991): 503–8.

7. Deborah Stone, *The Limits of Professional Power: National Health Care in the Federal Republic of Germany* (Chicago: University of Chicago Press, 1980).

8. Richard Wilkinson and Kate Pickett, *The Spirit Level: Why Greater Equality Makes Societies Stronger* (New York: Bloomsbury Press, 2009).

9. Tsung-Mei Cheng, "Understanding the 'Swiss Watch' Function of Switzerland's Health System," *Health Affairs* 29 (August 2010): 1442–51.

10. Ewout van Ginneken, Katherine Swartz, and Philip Van der Wees, "Health Insurance Exchanges in Switzerland and the Netherlands Offer Five Key Lessons for the Operations of US Exchanges," *Health Affairs* 32 (April 2013): 744–52.

11. David Himmelstein, Miraya Jun, Richard Busse, Karine Chevreul, Alexander Geissler, and Patrick Jeurissen, "A Comparison of Hospital Administrative Costs in Eight Nations: US Costs Exceed All Others by Far," *Health Affairs* 33 (September 2014): 1586–94.

12. Ellen Nolte and C. Martin McKee, "Measuring the Health of Nations: Updating an Earlier Analysis," *Health Affairs* 27 (January/February 2008): 58–71.

13. Commonwealth Fund, "Health Care Around the World: How Much Do You Know?" (January 23, 2015), http://www.commonwealthfund.org/publications/newsletters/the-commonwealth-fund-connection/2015/jan-26-2015/recent-releases/health-care-around-the-world.

14. Peter Hussey, Gerard Anderson, Robin Osborn, Colin Feek, Vivienne McLaughlin, John Millar, and Arnold Epstein, "How Does the Quality of Care Compare in Five Countries?" *Health Affairs* 23 (May/June 2004): 89–99.

8. HEALTH CARE REFORM: IS IT WORKING?

1. Teresa Coughlin, Sharon Long, Lisa Clemens-Cope, and Dean Resnick, "What Difference Does Medicaid Make?" Kaiser Family Foundation Reports, Urban Institute, May 2013.

2. Sue Ducat and Amy Martin Vogt, "National Health Spending Growth in 2013, at 3.6 Percent, Continued a Pattern of Low Growth for Five Consecutive Years," January 2015, http://contenthealthaffairs.org/lookup/doi/10.1377/hlthaff.2014.1107.

3. U.S. Department of Health and Human Services, "Efforts to Improve Safety Result in 1.3 Million Fewer Patient Harms, 50,000 Lives Saved and $12 Billion in Health Spending Avoided," December 2, 2014.

4. Benjamin Sommers, Katherine Baicker, and Arnold Epstein, "Mortality and Access to Care Among Adults After State Medicaid Expansion," *New England Journal of Medicine* 367 (September 2012): 1025–34.

5. John Wennberg and Alan Gittelsohn, "Variations in Medical Care," *Scientific American* 246 (April 1982): 120–34.

6. Michael Carome, "Sunshine Law Exposes Vast Industry Payments to Physicians," *Worst Pills, Best Pills News* 20 (December 2014): 2.

7. Gilbert Welch, Lisa Schwartz, and Steven Woloshin, *Overdiagnosed* (Boston: Beacon Press, 2011).

8. Shannon Brownlee, *Overtreated* (New York: Bloomsbury Press, 2007).

9. "Money-Driven Medicine: Understanding America's Healthcare Crisis," California Newsreel.org, http://www.moneydrivenmedicine.org.

10. Amber Sabbatini, Brahmajee Nallamothu, and Keith Kocher, "Reducing Variation in Hospital Admissions from the Emergency Department for Low-Mortality Conditions May Produce Savings," *Health Affairs* 33 (September 2014): 1655–63.

11. Agency for Healthcare Research and Quality, "New Snapshots Show States Vary in Providing Quality Care," August 2009.

12. OECD, "Health at a Glance 2011: OECD Indicators, Why Is Health Spending in the United States So High?," http://www.oecd.org/unitedstates/49084355.pdf.

13. Elisabeth Rosenthal, "How the High Cost of Medical Care Is Affecting Americans," *New York Times*/CNN News Poll, December 18, 2014.

14. Rand Corporation, "Eliminating Subsidies for People to Buy Health Coverage Would Increase Premiums and Number of Uninsured," October 21, 2014.

15. Bernie DiJulio, Jamie Firth, and Mollyann Brodie, Kaiser Health Policy Tracking Poll, December 18, 2014.

16. Kevin Sack and Marjorie Connelly, "In Poll, Wide Support for Government-Run Health," *New York Times*, June 21, 2009.

17. Physicians' Working Group for Single-Payer National Health Insurance, "Proposal of the Physicians' Working Group for Single-Payer National Health Insurance," *Journal of the American Medical Association* 290 (August 13, 2003): 798–805.

18. Ibid.

19. David Himmelstein, Deborah Thorne, and Steffie Woolhandler, "Medical Bankruptcy in Massachusetts: Has Health Reform Made a Difference?" *American Journal of Medicine* 124 (March 2011): 224–28.

20. Steffie Woolhandler and David Himmelstein, "Paying for National Health Insurance—and Not Getting It," *Health Affairs* 21 (July 2002): 88–98.

21. Wilhelmine Miller, Elizabeth Richardson Vigdor, and Willard Manning, "Covering the Uninsured: What Is It Worth?" Health Affairs web exclusive (March 31, 2004): w4-157–67, http://content.healthaffairs.org/content/early/2004/03/31/hlthaff.w4.157.citation.

22. Bernie Sanders, "A Single-Payer System Makes Economic Sense," September 13, 2013, http://www.sanders.senate.gov/newsroom/must-read/a-single-payer-system-makes-economic-sense.

23. Bernie Sanders, "Obamacare Is a 'Good Republican Program,'" September 24, 2013, http://politicalticker.blogs.cnn.com/2013/09/24/bernie-sanders-obamacare-is-a-good-republican-program/.

24. "Bernie Sanders Got Republicans to Make His Argument for Universal Health Care," January 23, 2015, http://www.huffingtonpost.com/2015/01/23/bernie-sanders-universal-_n_6534526.html.

25. Cathy Schoen, Karen Davis, Sabrina How, and Stephen Schoenbaum, "U.S. Health System Performance: A National Scorecard," *Health Affairs* 25 (November 2006): w5457–w5475.

26. David Williams, Mark McClellan, and Alice Rivlin, "Beyond the Affordable Care Act: Achieving Real Improvements in Americans' Health," *Health Affairs* 29 (August 2010): 1481–88.

27. Grace Budrys, *Unequal Health: How Inequality Contributes to Health or Illness* (Lanham, MD: Rowman and Littlefield, 2010).

9. PROVOCATIVE QUESTIONS AND CHALLENGING EXERCISES

1. Marcia Angell, *The Truth About the Drug Companies* (New York: Random House, 2004).

2. Cynthia Cox, Rosa Ma, Gary Claxton, and Larry Levitt, "Sizing Up Exchange Market Competition," Kaiser Family Foundation, March 1, 2014, http://kff.org/health-reform/issue-brief/sizing-up-exchange-market-competition/.

3. "Private Health Insurance: Concentration of Enrollees Among Individual, Small Group, and Large Group Insurers from 2010 through 2013," GAO-15-101R, December 1, 2014, http://www.gao.gov/assets/670/667245.pdf.

4. Robert Evans, *Strained Mercy: The Economics of Canadian Health Care* (Toronto: Butterworths, 1984).

INDEX

ABOUT THE AUTHOR

Grace Budrys is professor emerita at DePaul University, where she was a member of the Department of Sociology. Earlier in her academic career she served as director of the Public Services Master Program. More recently she chaired the committee charged with creating the Master of Public Health Program at DePaul University and served as director of the program. After receiving her doctorate at the University of Chicago she worked in a number of different health care organizations, including a university teaching hospital, a nonprofit dedicated to overcoming a leading cause of mortality, and a hospital consulting firm. Her writing reflects her interests and experiences. Her most recent books include *How Nonprofits Work* and *Unequal Health*, now in its second edition. This, the fourth edition of *Our Unsystematic Health Care System*, details the latest stage in the ongoing transformation of U.S. health care arrangements.